The Potent Immune-System Prevented my Cold/Flu

(Subtitle -**THE GLORIES AND PERILS OF SUPPLEMENTS**)
Erased My 33 Chronic Diseases and probably cancer

(Supplements: Herbal drugs, probiotics, Paleo diet, health and wellness life-styles, vitamins, minerals, essential oils, my own stem cells, Tiger Balms and home remedies).

"Glories" (of experimentations): 33 of my chronic diseases cured:
:Prevented: *Winter colds*
:Could prevent :*Heart attacks and strokes, my colon cancer
(Chapter 13) and other cancers* (Chapter 1)
:Cured: *Impotence. Allergies. Disabling arthritis. Benign Prostatic Hypertrophy. Six pounds lighter naturally, My white hair, black . Herpes zoster - shingles, cured instantly at the rash stage with an essential oil, on contact and more. All 33 ailments cured and described in this book.*

"Perils": *Increased chance of getting cancers from over-dosing (OD) and superfluous supplements. OD could lead to the ultimate peril of Death.*

"Immune potency maintenance"
Health and wellness habits of enough sleep, exercise and other knowledge that this book described, are necessary for immune system maintenance. Otherwise, it will lose the potency, which then becomes eroded.

Manuscripts of learnt self-experimentations by:
James C. Shum, M.D.

"Friendly Reminders" from a near-fatal Experience

I hate to use the authoritative word "warnings". So I replaced it with the more respectful words "friendly reminders", but the seriousness remains the same that herbs can be very dangerous.

Some books when giving advices on using (safe) herbs give the impressions that all side-effects of herbal drugs are mild. Indeed, the safe ones are. But in the real world, there are dangerous herbs just like there are dangerous medications. In fact, you can find a list of three dozen or so dangerous herbs in publications like the Mayo Clinic Book of Alternative Medicine. And if you want to know more about dangerous herbs, in the book PDR for Herbal Medicine, you can find hundreds of dangerous herbs. The word PDR stands for Physicians' Desk Reference.

One of the herbs listed in herbal PDR is *Ephedra*. It is used in the conventional medication called Pseudoephedrine which is an allergy drug. *Ehpedra* is dangerous.

I had a scary encounter with this California *Ephedra* plant. You see, I took seven pieces from the tips of the needle-shaped leaves. I thought this little pinch of leaves was a small dose. At the time, I was having sneezes, tears, and a runny nose when I was walking along the banks of a small river in the University of California at Davis (UC Davis). The plant was there by the roadside. It seemed willing and eager to help the miserable me. So I chewed and swallowed the *Ephdra* tips. My nasal allergy stopped in three minutes. My nose and eyes dried up. I was happy and grateful for the plant. It appeared just in time. I had only one piece of tissue left. It clearly was not enough for the copious amount of runny nose fluids. "Ha, I'm alright now", I thought, with a deep sigh of relief.

But a few seconds later, I experienced a big scare when I felt my heart skipped three beats! Those were strong beats that rocked my chest wall. That was really a big scare. If I took a few more tips of the leaves of *Ephedra*. My heart could have stopped as a side effect of overdosing on *Ephedra*. Lethal arrhythmia (irregular heart-beats) is known as one of the side effects of *Ephedra* per herbal PDR. And I could have been dead and became one of the mortality (death) figures of over-dosing on *Ephedra*. Many people died from overdosing when they used *Ephedra* for body-building or losing weight.

So when in one year in which seven people died of overdosing on Ephedra in the United States, it was banned totally. That was the year 2004. And it has been banned all over the world too.

With this encounter in my mind, I feel like a lucky survivor. I earnestly urge you to discuss with a knowledgeable health-care professional before committing yourself to taking any herbs. He or she would know whether your liver can handle the herbs, whether your kidneys can eliminate the herbs etc. (And to protect your kidneys from concentrated urines of toxins and the like, it is advisable to drink about eight tall glasses of water daily to dilute the chemicals in the urine, given people with normal kidneys and heart functions). So your kidneys won't get hurt.

It is my sincere hope that you can transform yourself into a very good healthy fellow like me, eliminated 33 chronic diseases as described in part 1 of this book. But before picking up any health-tips mentioned in this book, it is essential and necessary to run it by a health professional, for your own safety. Thank you indeed.

Disclaimer

There are many new studies and findings about good foods, bad foods and good life-styles in chapter 39. It ran 32 pages long. It is a whole lot of information of new sciences. Learning them all would transform your health for the better. To learn them easily is to read them now and then so the memory would stay. So take the book along for doctor's visits, for your vacation just to see repeatedly what new sciences have been found. In time, the health information will be ingrained in your brain and probably will benefit you like what they have benefited me. All my 33 chronic diseases are cured or well-controlled. Of course this does not constitute a promise from me. Everybody is different biologically. But most probably you will benefit.

Please make sure to consult your own health care professional before copying things I have done. As a medical doctor, I feel this is the appropriate request for you, so it can be safe for you. Food works wonders as Hippocrates, the Father of Medicine, said, "Food is medicine". After knowing the information well, and you know how to choose good foods, avoiding bad foods, then you probably can choose foods on your own. But if the foods are new to you, it is important to make sure the foods are not sensitive for you, even if they are good foods. Allergy doctors do have ways to find out and confirm your sensitivities to foods.

But for herbal medications, or even simple vitamins or other supplements, it does need a knowledgeable professional to check for drug interactions, contra-indications, to make sure it is safe for you.

For endurance exercise and high intensity exercises, most of us would need a doctor's advice. As for the 33 chronic diseases I cured myself of, some of it involved using herbs.

These reports remain accounts of experimentation. It has not been put through rigorous clinical trials. So it remains an experimental account, not a medical advice or recommendations. If you have the same chronic diseases and need symptomatic treatments, go see your doctor. But hopefully, the good foods that you are not allergic to, consumed regularly, may control the symptoms. Because to eat the good foods may just help you make the chronic diseases disappear, along with the symptoms. This is a distinct probability. It only takes two to four weeks to find out if that is the case for you.

But dangers can come from foods too, because some good foods can be allergic to some people. Like sea foods infrequently cause shock and death in some sensitive people. This kind of news is rare. But it does appear in newspapers when it happens. So make sure you are not allergic to the "good foods" before consuming them.

Also, when chronic diseases are thought to be "cured" and the alertness of avoiding bad foods are forgotten, makes one enjoy too many bad foods for a significant time would let the chronic diseases come right back.

Last, but not the least, herbal drugs that are deemed safe, even by the government, may still cause serious unexpected side effects. Take for example *Echinacea,* is generally considered a safe drug. But there were cases of liver or kidney failures associated with it. This reaction does happen to very rare unfortunate people. Start taking herbs under the guidance of a professional will be the advice.

Addendum to disclaimer – The disclaimer is extended to include a few words about a possible new flu virus in the future years. Vaccination is the only sure measure. Also there are a few words on cancer prevention.

Quite likely, with the information to maintain the potency of the immune system in this book, I would think my immune system may be able to defend me against any viral infection greatly. I hope it's true. But this is far from proven though it prevented my cold/flu for two years. There is always a small chance that Murphy's Law would apply. That is to say, if there is a 0.01% chance I could be infected with a new flu virus and die of it. I would die of it. This is Murphy's Law - If the worst could happen, it will happen. Yes, I hate Murphy's Law but I respect it.

So the best policy is still to avoid exposure to the flu infected people and to have flu-vaccination yearly.

As cancer prevention is concerned, this book expressed what I observed in my patients. It does not constitute medical advices or treatment recommendations. It remains a hypothesis till proven by large studies of randomized, double-blind, placebo-controlled studies undergone peer reviews. In other words, cancers can still occur even doing all findings from this book.

<u>CONTENTS</u>   **Page**

PART ONE

The Ailments I healed myself using Supplements mainly

<u>Chapters</u>

Part Two -- New Sciences

<u>Chapters</u>

Part Three -- Prevention with New Sciences
Chapters

Part Four – Interesting Matters
Chapters

Proclamation: It's easy to transform your health and save the healthcare cost in USA.

You may think it is difficult for you to do for such great things. But it is not exactly difficult how I transformed myself into a person who is healthier with a well-oiled immune system. The strengthened immune system enabled me to avert the winter cold I got yearly and I hope it will help me to fend off the Respiratory virus pandemic. And I became stronger physically with a faster metabolism to burn off fat---six pounds lighter. I became smarter with no more brain fog. Better recent memory and shredded the absent-minded professor habits a lot. That was quite a transformation to good health. And all it needs is just doing one thing which I called "one smart-move". It is so simple you may not believe it. It is to avoid bad foods which got rid of my 33 chronic diseases.

The transformation started not too long ago. In fact, it was about a year and a half ago when I learned how to get rid of my erectile dysfunction, brain fog, disabling arthritis, yearly "cold", absent-mindedness and a total of about thirty-three chronic ailments.

Before that, I was strong in the past, now I am *stronger and healthier*. If most people transform themselves and get rid of their chronic diseases. The healthcare cost in USA may be plummeted and then we can avoid virtual bankruptcy by the year 2040. By then, the cost of healthcare is estimated to be equal to the National Taxation Income. If the healthcare takes every penny we produced, we would have no money left for the rest of the country. Isn't that virtual bankruptcy?

What did I do to rid myself of chronic disease like diarrhea, brain fog, mental deterioration with aging, and stay young (anti-aging) and more? Besides the "one smart move" I did, it is just plus some old lifestyle habits.

So first, let me go back to a little earlier to what kept me physically young and strong, but with a slight brain-fog, and a slightly weak immune system allowing a mild cancer "attack" 16 years ago? Though, at that time, I thought it had been good enough. Just imagine, for four decades I religiously do my routine exercise that kept me and my wife looking young and strong. In our ages of 70's, we look like in our 50's. This has been good physically, but it did nothing to the chronic diseases mentioned above and more, like skin looking ugly, mood swings could pop up. These chronic diseases I learned to get rid off after retirement.

Exercise is not enough for my transformations. But exercise was the only things needed, for some folks? For whom? For my patients I was taking care of before retirement. They were patients treated for cancers of various kinds. Most of them are still alive even now almost ten years later. The patients learned seven cancer fighting habits from me, one of them is exercise. They avoided cancer coming back more than patients who did not have the life-style knowledge I gave my patients that information beyond standard treatments.

I was a medical oncologist before retirement. I found a few cancer fighting methods from pure scientific studies to augment standard cancer treatments. After my patients took from me a full page of notes on seven smart life-styling habits, they built themselves up physically, and mentally, with a stronger immune system than before, feeling good to be able to have found more ways to fight cancer besides the traditional treatment methods. They got the gifts of new lives, or years longer to live. (The ones with *early stage* cancers never saw cancer coming back. Normally 30% patients with early cancers, the cancer would come back. The ones with *late-stage* cancers survived three to five years while similar patients in the real world last one year or so).

What were those seven earlier smart life-style habits? They were great in helping conventional cancer treatments:

1. *Appropriate amount of exercise. 2. Eat 80% full, never eat till full. And if hunger strikes between meals, eat nuts, seeds, or dark chocolate. 3. Get rid of stress. 4. Absolutely no sugar. 5. Keep the same weight.* 6. Eat plenty of non-starchy vegetables. 7. Adequate sleep of 6 to 8 hours a day. These seven golden habits that I gave to patients were written on a single piece of paper, with explanations extracted from research studies. Together with standard therapies, they dwarfed cancers. They have been the reason of my eternal delight.

It is about to get even better. Because there is another "one smart move" that may involve seven more smart lifestyle tips to foster a stronger immune system, better mental health and getting rid of more than 33 of my chronic diseases. I never learned these in medical school in New York in the 1970's. This is from new sciences I studied after retirement. The seven newer habits consisted of 4 foods to avoid because they are inflammatory; and three diet habits to form. It will be explained fully in chapter 39.

These seven tips I learned after researching through herbal medicine trying to find herbs that can enhance the immune system. I do not think I found any. Then, chronic inflammation caught my attention. Newer science discovered inflammation is the cause of chronic diseases like strokes, heart attacks, cancers, and in fact, all chronic disease including auto-immune diseases. There is a chapter on inflammation and diseases, in chapter 42. To reduce inflammation, is to calm down the immune system, as described in chapter one. Yes, all these have been "proven" in studies.

Then I found out the best means of calming down the immune system. It is simply not to bring in outside enemies that greatly out-number our immune cells. So it is important to shut down the gates letting these enemies in. It is to shut tight the leaky gut.

These studies brought me to more new sciences about the gut bacteria. There are tons of research on gut bacteria now, they call it gut microbiota or microbiome. These bacteria evolved with us over millions of years and became part of our virtual organ systems. They have gene mass 173 times more than ours. Most of the bacterial genes were found to make pre-hormones or pre-chemicals for our body to convert and use. The microbiome is a chemical factory for us in practicality.

And the gut bacteria ask for very little. They just need us to eat the right foods and avoid the wrong foods. That led to the studies of Paleo diet, Mediterranean diets and finally, I found the golden key that opened the door to the good health I am enjoying now.

But if I were to take only two of the above 14 beneficial habits, I will take exercise and the Paleo-like diet, or Mediterranean-like diet. They were extensively studied. They are very potent means of strengthening our body's immune systems and enlightening our mind. All my myriad of 33 chronic diseases that I conquered as described in Part One of this book, would not have been happened in the first place, only if I had known these tips when I was young. They are real *Chronic Disease Terminators, eliminating all my chronic diseases.*

If we can emphasize all these *Chronic Disease Terminators* in medical schools and set up to educate the general public. In the long run, most citizens should become well-patients without chronic diseases. They would enjoy better and healthier lives. Caring for them would be minimal effort required, and a lot less expensive.

Without the cost of chronic diseases economically burdening us, we'll be able to pay little health-care cents instead of big health-care dollars. This may save Uncle Sam from going broke in 2040 because of the escalating health-care cost. It has been estimated by the year 2040, the Health-care expense may be equal to our whole-nation taxation. Folks, are you ready to transform yourself? Be patriotic to save USA. If not, at least save your selves from most chronic diseases. It may only take two week to four weeks, then you may start to see results.

PART ONE

I healed 33 of my Ailments

(with Supplements mainly, plus smart lifestyle habits)

Chapter One - How I got rid of my yearly Cold by making my Immune System potent.

Introduction

I spent 53 years to find the cause and cure of cancer. After 20 years of my pursuit, I became convinced that a weakness in the immune system allowed the cancer to start. But what caused the weakness in the immune system? I kept on searching.

Hundreds of research papers provided seven smart lifestyles that improve the immune system to fight cancer from population studies. I adapted them for my patients. As a result of my patients practicing the smart lifestyles, most seemed to have gotten free from cancer recurrence and others lived years longer. Primary care colleagues became aware of their unexpected long lives and were aware their patients always appeared in the follow up, (and not dead yet). And medical records of my patients showed lack of recurrences and prolonged survivals.

Finally by year 53, I found everything I could to keep the immune system potent. That will be discussed in this chapter and the rest of the book which is about how to make the immune system potent. And most chapters described the bonus for me to be fee from more than 30 chronic diseases.

That is what this book is all about.

I suffered from mild cold/flu almost every winter after I retired from the job of a specialist physician (Hematologist/oncologist). For seven winters, I routinely got a cold which were all very mild. But after I have learned the final new sciences of keeping my immune system potent for the past 2 years, I have been free of winter cold/flu. I will elaborate on the new sciences of keeping the immune system potent in this chapter. I did live by those sciences as you can see. But I understand some facts remain empirical, not all of them were proven by "golden studies", but most findings are from good studies.

Strengthened my immune system against Cancer

I hope you can have some patience to finish this chapter, then you understand how I restored a strong immune system, never getting a cold in the winter. That was 2 years before this pandemic. With this restored immune system, I hope I will prevent a colon cancer which I have 8 times more risk. The potent immune system may give me a better chance to survive this respiratory virus pandemic which is an infection just like a cold. But no one should take the chance of depending only on a potent immune system. But it is easier on the mind when we know the infection seems to be a mild one and we have some ways to make the immune system potent. It is good to let panic go.

Panic is equal to worry. It is bad. Being panicky can weaken your immune system, so says the studies. So you do have to read this long chapter to know more about keeping the immune-system potent and how to strengthen your immune system for the life-battle and hopefully to prevent cancers too, because I studied to make the immune system potent for fighting cancers.

At the end of this chapter, there are a few more scientific paragraphs of maintaining the potency of the immune system to prevent cancers (and perhaps able to fight the Respiratory virus pandemic). So please read on. No immune-potency-maintenance is no good. We got to learn it.

How to keep the immune system potent – Introduction:

After 53 years of seeking the most potent immune system for my patients to fight cancers. I succeeded in 30 years. I found some lifestyles actions to make immune systems potent. With those measures my more than 600 patients prevented cancer from coming back when they have early stage cancers. The patients with late stage cancers extended their survival by 3 to 5 years more. This is a phenomenal number if you consider their survival should just be counted in terms of months.

I will list the seven lifestyles that dwarfed cancers soon. But I have been practicing those lifestyles too, yet despite practicing these lifestyles, I still got a desmoids tumor around that time 16 years ago. Desmoid tumor is really a low grade cancer in the sarcoma category. So there was more to immune potency I was missing. It let a cancer start and grow.

It was the erosion of immune-potency that I missed. The knowledge of immune potency erosion I only had a chance to learn after I retired. I spent about two years to read about 1500 pages of herbal medicine and did not find herbs that help keep the immune system potent, at least not when taken on short term. I looked elsewhere.

Started two years ago, I started to read a dozen books written by Functional Medicine gurus, most of them physicians. Then I had to read what they base their wonderful healing power on. They emphasized gut health, probiotics (good bacteria in our gut), and good foods and bad foods on top of healthy lifestyles.

I was skeptical. After all, it was simply avoiding bad foods and any allergens that could end up weakening the immune system, they say. But all of those functional medicine physicians swear they had cured thousands of patients with autoimmune diseases and chronic diseases due to internal inflammation from eating bad foods.

Another year and a half of reading extensively on the above topics, and at the same time, I experimented on myself with what I learned from them. At the end, I was dumbfounded. It really worked. More than 30 of my chronic diseases evaporated. I feel like a different person with lightness of being, not on any drugs for that matter.

What did the simple act of avoiding bad foods and eating good foods did to me? I gave it a lot of deep mental analysis. Then I realized what this magic bullet of functional medicine treatment is. It is to avoid "immune potency erosion". The evaporation of the chronic diseases is just the bonus. My yearly winter cold has stopped for two years. Avoiding immune-potency-erosion to achieve immune potency is the real key harvest.

I will list the immune-potency erosions soon.

So to have a potent immune system, I need to boost the immune system as well as avoiding eroding its potency. Both are necessary and almost sufficient to keep the immune system potent.

First let's look at the immune boosting lifestyles that were shown to prevent cancer coming back for 600 of my patients. There were expected to have at least 100 recurrences (Cancers coming back) in the ten years before my retirement when the patient learned all the seven survival tips I gave them on a piece of paper. Really I hardly remembered any recurrence of cancer coming back. Immune-potency boosting indeed are truly useful. These lifestyles I extracted from about 500 research papers.

I will elaborate more on exercise and calorie restriction after the seven items are listed as follows.

The seven smart life-style actions that dwarfed cancers by boosting immune potency are:

.Exercise: Long known to enhance the immune system. It boosts immune system by various means. It was all from studies. The underlying sciences were elaborated in my other books (sold at cost, and can be ordered on line by typing my name down in Google search).

.Eat till 80% full: It takes 20 minutes for an already full stomach to tell the brain to stop eating. If you eat till full. You eat too much and would gain weight. Gaining weight in studies was shown to weaken the immune system. On the other hand, active weight-loss strengthens the immunity. The best is to eat till 80% full and drink a cup of fluid to make it a 100% full, and eat nuts if really hungry later (if there is no allergy to nuts). Just a handful of nuts are enough. It has very high calories. It is easy to over eat nuts.

.Relieve stress: Stress increase inflammation in our body. Blood test will show the inflammation with stress. Inflammation-stress weakens the immune system. Sleep-deprivation (less than 5 hours of sleep) is the number one reason for stress in America according to studies. It lowers the immune potency right away besides causing stress. Stress hormone prednisone suppresses the lymphocytes and antibody producing cells (white blood cells) of the immune system. When stress is released, the immune potency is regained. Studies showed that less than 5 hours sleep can weaken the immune system by 70% (Less NK cells – important immune white blood cells).

.No sugar – It is very inflammatory and immune-potency eroding. Americans eat the most calories from sugar, from Tuft University study. The sugar is in the form of high fructose corn syrup (HFCS) in all processed foods. Why is it bad? HFCS is main reason for getting us fat and for fatty liver disease. Sugar is also the only fuel for cancer cells.

.Keep the same weight (i.e. don't gain weight). Weight gain is gaining fats. Fat cells make inflammatory chemicals. Inflammation weakens the immune system. So avoid eating saturated fats.

    To keep the same weight, I had to do regular exercises and do my calorie restriction (Eating till 80% full). So maintaining a stand weight is essential.

.Eat a lot of vegetables – Only after retirement I got the chance to learn the benefit of what I advised, that eat a lot of vegetables means a lot of fibers that eventually heal the gut and enhance the immune potency. That will be explained more later on. But eating a lot of vegetables was one of the advices I gave before retirement to patients. At that time, we had not learned that fibers are good foods for the gut bacteria that repair a leaky gut, and enhance our immune system function.

.Avoid red meats – That was also one of the advice I gave. The advice was chosen from past studies. New sciences now showed red meats with saturated fats could be inflammatory. Studies showed also if eaten with lots of fibers or omega-3 rich food, the saturated fats can be anti-inflammatory too. That means half a plate of non-starchy vegetables.

Emphasizing the importance of exercise:
A sure way to boost your immune potency, exercise saved lives and even can prevent cancers the first time or for cancers coming back

Unassuming as they have been, the smart life-styling listed above, however, has really been the essence of reports from hundred-million-dollars studies like the Nurses Health Study (NHS). It showed statistically nurses who have cancers but continue to do regular exercises, their survival is 50% better. This is not the only study showing exercises save lives. There are a few dozen biggie studies like the Health Professionals Follow Up Study, Women's Health Initiative and more. They all showed it can prevent primary cancer (lowered the risk of cancer) by 40%, prevent cancer recurrence of also 40% and increased survival after cancer treatment by 50%.

So there is no wonder more than 500 of my patients with early stage cancer seemed never recurred. I expected about 100 cancer recurrences, but I hardly remembered any. So this clinical experience gives me the peace of mind, that even when I have eight times the risk of colon cancer due to irritable bowel syndrome, and there was a polyp in my last colonoscopy (Polyps are fore-runners of colon cancer, for 100% of the colon cancers), I think I still can beat the odds. I just have to keep up my exercises and not to over-exercise.

The next I am going to emphasize is calorie restriction.

Calorie Restriction, eating till 80% full is important

When we feel full at dinners, we are actually eating a full 120% if it is vegetable mainly good diet. If we eat a high percentage of good fats which are also good diets, and if we eat till feeling full, it would be 140%, because the good fats have doubled the calories. No matter, overeating is right there when we feel full, because the stomach will not give the message to the brain when it is really full. It gives the signal only twenty minutes later according to very old studies. That is why it is important to stop before feeling a little full and drink a cup of liquids to distend the stomach to give the feeling of fullness.

This is important for immune potency and cancer control. Let me first show one case of a carcinoid tumor (Meaning a little cancer) disappeared in one of my patients who did strict calorie restriction (CR) and lost 3 pounds. And then I will show you two cases of my patients giving up on CR for a couple of weeks almost die of the diseases. All 3 were my patients.

Emphasizing eating till 80% full, case # 1
Calorie restrictions to control cancer

Thanks to the same (old) smart habits, one of my patients did have her carcinoid (means a little cancer) eliminated from her left lung. She did not want surgery for the golf-ball size carcinoid in her left lower lung. I gave her the information for the seven lifestyle actions listed above. There is no good chemotherapy for it either.

For months, she worked hard at those habits and lost 3 pounds by 6 months follow up. (This case was described in my other books). She restored her immune potency with the smart life-styling. The smart habits mainly of calorie restriction enabled her to shred 3 pounds.

By 6 months follow-up, a CT (Computer tomography) showed the golf-ball size carcinoid tumor disappeared from her lung. Her immune system improved enough to get rid of the "little cancer", the carcinoid tumor. Most such tumors are slow growing. But rare ones can be rapidly fatal. It did not matter to her. It was gone. And she knew what good lifestyle actions to do to keep it away.

A good immune system is enough to prevent cancer recurrence or even get rid of a "little cancer" so far. It is capable to prevent cancer in the first place from the above life experiences of my patients (not from studies).

Emphasizing eating till 80% full case # 2
Patient with myelocysplastic syndrome (MDS) who survived because of strictly living with "eating till 80% full" (The management was empirical but very effective)

Next is going to be a case of an elderly male who is a prominent member of the society. He had a disease of "making no blood cells", or making very little blood cells. He was not a bone marrow transplant candidate. With low platelets, which are a small blood "cells", he could bleed to death. Platelet transfusion won't work after a few transfusions when his immune system would destroy the platelets given, (the platelets were collected from other people). Or his low white blood cells could get him fatal infections anytime. But with some molecular drug treatments, he was able to maintain a decent white blood counts and platelet levels after he practiced the lifestyle actions listed above, including calorie restrictions. That lasted a miraculous 3 years before I retired.

Once he went to England to meet some friends, liberated his calories restrictions, he came back in the hospital, bleeding. He feasted for two weeks in England. CR rescued him and I had to add a second molecular drug. We did not know why his disease worsened at that time. Only after later, he drove up from Northern California to Michigan to meet friends and feasted again. He had bleeding again when he came back. But spontaneously recovered with the same two molecular drugs, and the obedient-student like diet of CR rescued him. Only then, we realized it was the joyful feasting both times that got him bleeding because of low platelets.

If he was not a compliant patient who practiced the above lifestyles, and the diseases called myelocysplastic syndrome, MDS, could get out of control. He would surely die either of bleeding or infection in a year or two.

Calorie-restrictions besides cured a little-cancer and stopping a clone of cells that can mess up the bone marrow in the MDS case as we discussed above, actually has a key role in achieving disease controls of cancer. It also lowers internal inflammations in studies. The key role of calorie restriction is in preventing weight gain. Keeping the same weight is hard to do. But eating till 80% full would be the key to help.

I have a 3rd case to illustrate the great harm of forgoing calorie-restriction and feeding cancer cells with more sugar.

Emphasizing eating till 80% full case # 3
A sad case of liberating calories and supplying enough sugar is detrimental to cancer control

Sugar is very inflammatory, and hurts the immune potency. This will be emphasized again and again in later chapters. And over-calorie for cancer is detrimental. The case in focus is an end stage liver cancer that is very hard to treat.

I never forget what a night of nutrition including high sugar could do to cancer. One of my patients was a young lady. She underwent tough chemotherapy that needed to be given in the hospital. She wanted to soften her liver cancer so she could live longer at least till all her relatives could come from all over the world to visit. After chemotherapy in the hospital for 5 days, her liver cancer became so soft I could not feel them anymore. One night of intravenous nutrition that has high sugar in it (The right thing to do for a very thin patient). The liver cancer grew back rock-hard. I almost cried, after examining the patient the morning of discharge. After that case, I became a stern believer in avoiding sugar even for normal people.

She went home, was able to last six weeks when she resumed calorie restriction. Hopefully that was enough time for her to see all her relatives from all over the world.

With cancer control, I always emphasize on calorie restriction. But extreme calorie restriction on long term for weight-control could lead to under-nutrition and weakens the immune system. But it is different in practicing eating till feeling 80% full. It is actually 100% full because the delay in the message delivered to the brain from the stomach when it is full. The delay is 20 minutes.

Appropriate calorie restriction can lower the internal inflammation as in studies. Lowering the internal inflammation is going to make the immune system more potent.

Other measures to keep the immune system potent:

Besides the above seven measures listed to keep the immune system potent, there are a few more things I do. All of the measures are shown by studies, they will be elaborated in the chapters that will follow especially chapter 39. I am just going to list them briefly in this chapter.

1. Multivitamins, vitamins C, D, E. I take them because the foods have been grown in depleted soils. That is the advice of most health gurus.
2. I take *Korean ginseng.* It is a popular adaptogen that decreases the stress of life, improves stamina. It has been taken by humans for thousands of years. The *Korean ginseng* has more stimulating effects than the *American ginseng* or *Siberian ginseng* which are calming in effects.
3. Paleo, vegetarian, or Mediterranean diets till feeling 80% full plus a cup of liquids. The food items in them are anti-inflammatory.
4. Probiotics are living bacteria in our gut, supposed to represent good bacteria. It was proven to enhance immunity. It will be discussed again and again in this book, and in chapter 39. There is initial evidence that it does increase immune potency, but needs more studies. The only worry I have is when persons with severely compromised immunity, is it safe to take? I am not sure. I would hesitate to say yes to people with weak immune systems to take probiotics. After all, these are bacteria.

The immune boosting effects of the above measures are all from studies. They showed effectiveness in hundreds of my patients avoiding cancer recurrences. It left me no doubt they are real effective measures for a potent immune system. They passed the test of real life effectiveness and saved 1 to 2 hundreds of my patients from cancer recurrences which may mean eventually leading to deaths from recurrent cancers.

So I wish to express thanks to the thousands of researchers that produced those hundreds of papers I read while working as an oncologist mainly in California, for saving these lives.

Those are immune boosting measures. But it was not enough for me. I got a low grade sarcoma at the beginning of that time period. So there was something more that I needed to keep the immune system potent. For eight years after I retired, involved readings failed to reveal what were missing that actually weakened my immune system without me knowing it, till I learned it at last in the last two years or so. It is erosion of the immune potency.

I will list about five such life-habits that lead to the weakening by immune erosion. For the leaky gut syndrome, exhaustive exercising and sleep deprivation, I will provide explanations or examples. For other life habits that hurt the immune system, like smoking and excessive alcohol consumption. They are well-known by everybody. I am just going to list them.

Actions (life habits) that erodes the Immune Potency: The followings are some common reasons:

1. Leaky gut syndrome is affecting millions of people. It includes me. A lively case will be discussed from reading of one of the books (6). Leaky gut allowed a cancer in a 3-years old girl to grow and later her healing the leaky gut, cured the cancer.

    I stopped my irritable bowel syndrome, my chronic diseases went away, and it prevented my yearly winter cold/flu for two years in a row now. So avoiding erosion of my immune potency, I got the normal and potent immune system that prevented colds/flu for me. (Vaccination is really the right thing to do, but needle and I are not in good terms).

2. Sleep-deprivation – examples are doctors and nurses and other health professionals who died due to sleep-deprivation in the current viral respiratory pandemic, I think.

3. Other habits like smoking, excessive alcohol consumption and obesity.

4. Low fat diet leading to obesity. That will be discussed again and again in different chapters. Low fat diets are rejected by all health gurus and authors nowadays. The infamous food pyramid contained too much carbohydrate (Not specifying what is "good carb" or "bad carb" at that time) that the liver converts to fat. It leads to the astronomical increase in over-weight, obesity and fatty liver diseases.

5. Endurance exercises and over strenuous exercise were found in studies to weaken the immune potency for 4 to 6 hours immediately after. In that period of times, people get respiratory infections easier. That is why it is recognized swimmers get winter colds and other respiratory infections easier and often.

Emphasizing Leaky Gut Syndrome eroding immune potency

I will present a case to illustrate this. New science: **The strongest way to enhance your immune system: Restore its potency. Analysis from an actual case.**

Hold on to your seat belts now. I will describe a case I read from a book (6) with a fatal cancer spontaneously disappeared. I will try to explain the scientific events of the immune system that helped the patient with some hypothesis. The patient, a 3-year old little girl who restored her immune system by improving her gut health, and her restored immune system resumed its normal potency and got rid of a fatal cancer. The case was an actual case probably presented in an opthalmology grand-round in a hospital. The case was well publicized in books and on the "web" about the event. Here in this book, I will try to hypothesize the immunological events that make this possible.

You can read the case in the internet if you can find it. It is also very well described in Dr Tom O'Bryn's book (6). The case was a 3 year old named Molly in the book. She was found to have Kaposi's sarcoma in her right eye. The cancer would be fatal. At the same time, she had a leaky gut wall and a damaged small intestinal mucosa in the disease called celiac disease. The damage is due to allergy to foods containing gluten. Her immune system was weakened by celiac disease in her small intestines.

Emphasizing Leaky Gut Syndrome eroding immune potency continues:

How did celiac disease weaken Molly's immune system to allow a fatal cancer to start? Let me hypothesize to understand the immune system related to strengthening.

She had leaky gut walls as part of the Celiac Disease. This allowed millions and millions of very minute food particles and dead gut bacterial parts of protein, nucleic acid and others to enter into her circulation. These particles were foreign to her system. In time, there must be billions of dead bacterial parts. (It was analyzed and found out half of our bowel content are dead bacterial parts from the bacteria dying naturally, mainly in our colon). The total weight of the live and active bacteria is 3 to 5 pounds. Scientists called it gut microbiome or microbiota which have been with human beings for millions of years.

After being absorbed from her gut and into her circulation, the very tiny food particles and bacterial parts were regarded as foreign bodies. The immune system gets into action to attack those particles like attacking harmful bacteria, try to get rid of them, by secreting chemicals that are inflammatory to burn them dead. This happens all over her body in the circulation. Mind you, there were millions and millions of foreign bodies in every inch of her little body. Now there are billions and billions of chemicals secreted by the immune cells, those chemicals are inflammatory creating big time internal inflammation that would burn weak systems.

Is Molly's immune system capable of getting rid of that many foreign objects (antigens)? Absolutely not, I think as another proposition. The immune system evolved to fight local wars. This is my assumption or hypothesis as I could observe from experiences in my clinical years. It is only capable of killing all bacteria in an infected wound, a limited local area. That is a local war we all may win, like a common cold, which is localized to the upper respiratory tract in the nose and throat.

But if bacteria get into our blood and doubles itself every twenty minutes or so, they will circulate to every inch of our body. This generalized disease is now a world war. We then will have a definite chance of dying from this "world war" like infection. That is why a lot of patients died from bacteremia (bacterial infection in the blood stream) or sepsis even when treated with potent antibiotics in Intensive Care Units. This world war like infection we were not evolved to fight as I further hypothesize, again from clinical observations of people dying from such massive infections.

The leaky gut of Molly's Celiac disease brought her a world war. The immune system did not evolve to fight such wars.

The world war will never end unless her leaky gut is mended, stopping the agents that caused the war, the foreign particles. Before she mended her guts, the foreign particles outnumbered the immune cells, disabling her immune system, generating inflammatory immune-chemicals. Molly was in big trouble. The dysfunctional immune system could not stop the Kaposi's sarcoma from initiation and could grow and be fatal in weeks in her age-group.

Emphasizing Leaky Gut Syndrome eroding immune potency continues: Mend the leaky gut. Restore her immune system. Molly's immune system killed the Kaposi's sarcoma in her right eye (that, is the fact).

The dysfunctional system was all due to a leaky gut. Fortunately, this leakiness of the gut was reversible. Just avoid eating the wrong allergenic foods. Once the gut is not leaky when Molly stopped eating gluten containing foods, the bad foods I have been referring to, her guts shut tight. No more foreign objects like the dead bacterial parts could get in now. Her immune system was restored. By nature, her immune system recognized the Kaposi cells as foreign, labeled it and destroyed it slowly. Gradually, one by one, the cancer cells all died. What supports this point as a third hypothesis is from the collective experiences of the functional medicine professionals treating hundreds of thousands of their patients. Their findings was mending a leaky gut lower our inflammation and got rid of the chronic diseases in their patients, hundreds of thousands of them.

Cancer is regarded as a chronic disease.

Do I believe in mending the leaky guts improving my immune potency, and getting rid of my chronic diseases. Yes I do. And that is what the main content of this book is all about. The immune-system became so potent it prevented my winter colds/flu as I continued my endurance swimming. But how did I mend my leaky guts? That's next.

How I mend my leaky gut that erodes immune potency:#1. How can I mend a leaky gut and restore the potency of the immune system, this new science?

Eating foods like the Stone Age people ate, the Paleo diet (explained soon) will mend a leaky gut because it excluded the most important bad foods that most susceptible people are allergic to. (Allergies to foods caused leaky guts and poor immune system though we may not know it. Thus bad foods are dangerous to health).

Not only Paleo diets can be good. So can other diets like the Mediterranean diet or even vegetarian diets can mend a leaky gut too. That will get you the best immune system. The Old Stone Age diet is called the Paleo Diet, abbreviated from the word Paleolithic, the Old Stone Age. Those foods would lower your body's slow burning fire, the chronic inflammation that cause arthritis, cancer, heart attack and strokes. There will be a whole chapter (Chapter 42) on chronic inflammation in this book. It is the real silent killer.

How I mend my leaky gut that erodes immune potencyby mending the leaky gut with diets: # 2. What is the Paleo diet? What is Mediterranean diet?

To say briefly what the main theme of the Paleo diet is: It avoids inflammatory foods and eats anti-inflammatory foods. Eat foods that the Stone Age people ate, they are not inflammatory because their digestive systems (like most of ours) was evolved over millions of years to digest the foods. That excluded *milk, wheat, sugar and salt.* These foods came after the agricultural revolution that happened about ten thousand years ago. Our digestive system had evolved over millions of years ago, not evolved to digest these new foods. Also, eating good proteins, good fats, and good carbohydrates are important because they all can lower the internal inflammations, shown in studies.

Good proteins are the meats that are low in saturated fat, like chicken, fish, turkey, lean meats, grass-fed beef, free range chicken meat and eggs. Shell-fish, fish and other sea foods have good oils called omega-3.

Good carbohydrates are the ones that are not starchy. Examples of starchy foods are potato, sweet potatoes and too much grains.

Good fats include fatty fish, olive oil, olive, seeds and nuts, avocado, and dark chocolates, duck fats, coconut oils. Duct fats have more unsaturated fats.

The underlying sciences of why they are anti-inflammatory will be explained in Part Two - New Sciences in the chapter of "Good foods, Bad foods" in chapter 39.

Mediterranean diet is rich in fatty fish, olive, olive oil and lots of vegetables just similar to Paleo diet or vegetarian diet in some aspects.

How I mend my leaky gut that erodes immune potency:# 3. Milk and dairy products, wheat, flour and legumes, and grains. Are they really that bad?

I am not sure. Just because these items were not seen in the Old Stone Age archaeological finds, and with a small number of people allergic to gluten resulting in celiac disease or may be also Irritable

Bowel Syndrome, then flatly reject wheat and flour products as bad would sound unscientific. It needs study to say they are really bad for people. But gluten in wheat-products does harm the 5% of people who are so allergic to gluten that they develop celiac disease resulting in a lousy immune system like Molly's, should be called a terrible food. For 80% of people who are allergic to gluten to a lesser degree, eating too much definitely is also bad. (Gluten has been proven in humans to cause leaky gut because it induces zonulin which open up tight junctions in gut cells, making it leaky).

For processed foods, there is no doubt, it can cause internal inflammation. Studies have confirmed processed foods are bad. To me, they are "poisonous" yet are usually delicious. With high contents of sugar, fat and salt, they are all inflammatory. Any substance added to the processed food would taste good, when lots of sugar, salt and fats are there. But they are really bad.

In later modern archaeological finds, grains and nuts were present in the "New Stone Age" people. Though, I am sure you won't find milk or milk products in those archaeological finds as it was very hard to ask a husky primordial wild cow to stand still so the cavemen could milk them. And agricultural revolution came 10,000 years ago. From then to now, it has been ten thousand years passed, this prolonged length of time may allow gene-changes in some people. So to those people whose genes have changed, these nutritious foods may not be bad at all. Like 80% of Northern Europeans have the gene to digest milk, while 80% of Asians and African Americans cannot digest milk.

Genes-sets do change over time. An example is the seeds of a Judean date palm tree from the ancient Israeli fortress of Masada about 2000 years ago. A modern scientist germinated the 2000 years old seed. A date palm tree grew from the ancient seed from two thousand years ago. The tree looks like a modern date palm tree. But it only has 50% of the genes identical to the modern date palm trees. Half the total genes are different in 2000 years. Science says animal genes could change the same with time.

**How I mend my leaky gut that erodes immune potency:#
4. Genes could have changed to make bad foods good**

So there should be a significant percentage of people whose genes could have changed and could tolerate the new foods in town that came after the agricultural revolution ten thousand years ago. Those foods are milk, wheat and flour products, salt and sugar. But you would never have known how harmful they can be for you. Even though you think you can tolerate them, does not mean you are not allergic to them.

How I mend my leaky gut that erodes immune potency:# 5. How could we know if milk, bread and sugar or salt are causing us allergies and bad chronic diseases?

Stop these foods for two weeks to four weeks, and see if you have chronic diseases going away or not. If chronic diseases go away on stopping eating bread, milk and sugar, in two to four weeks, you know you are allergic, and your chronic diseases are the result. That include acne, and all 33 chronic diseases I had and more.

I believe in 10,000 years, some human genes could have evolved to digest the agricultural new foods. May not be all of us, but at least some of us. The foods there were not present in Paleolithic Age include wheat (Bread, cakes, cookies, and most processed foods), beans, grains, legumes, milk, sugar, and salt. So if your stomach does not feel well after ingesting these foods. Your genes probably have not evolved enough to digest those foods. It is better to avoid that particular food.

How I mend my leaky gut that erodes immune potency:# 6. Wheat and flour products and milk and milk products are bad ONLY for some

But I am not saying wheat, wheat product and milk would not cause sensitivity problems for *all* people. I am a good example. As for wheat and wheat products, I have found out I am sensitive to them. If I eat too much delicious bread, I would find acne on my face soon. Acne is a good indicator of worse inflammation in my body. That is because my deranged immune system due to bread (gluten) begins to" attack:" my hair follicles (more to discuss in the chapter on acne, Chapter 8). It goes away with anti-inflammatory foods. This may not work for all people but it's worth a trial. Everyone has different sensitivity to different foods. If you stop eating a particular food from the above list, your chronic diseases like arthritis, acne, acid reflux, upset stomach etc gets better, then you probably are sensitive to that food. Then these foods are so called "bad foods" for you.

How I mend my leaky gut that erodes immune potency:# 7. How about my taste bud problem with the new foods I don't used to like? Good question.

Give any foods two weeks. You will find any new foods become tasty. Why? In two weeks, your taste buds cells will all be renewed. The new cells like the new foods. And you will find the new foods delicious.

Emphasizing on sleep deprivation that erodes immune potency – The reason why more than 100 doctors and nurses died of the Coronaviral infection pandemic: Sleep deprivation.

With the Coronaviral pandemic of 2019-2020, more than 100 doctors and other professionals all over the world died. They were young, most of them. Why should young people die of viral respiratory infections? That was not the case with influenza infections in the past years? Is the virus more virulent? Probably not. Are the professionals that died weaker in the immune systems? Yes, even though only temporarily.

How do they got their immune system weakened? My experience in the AIDS epidemic may suggest an answer. It is sleep-deprivation. When HIV infection first started in the early 1980's, it was totally unknown. And nobody knew it suppressed the immune system and caused pneumonia by pneumocystis carinii. So I remembered running numerous tests day and night just to find out why these young patients kept on dying due to pneumonias. Almost every night when on call, I never stopped running. I had no chance to sit. It was running all night to take care of the AIDS patients, to do tests, or to do resuscitations on another AIDS young patient dying, several times a night sometimes. A few weeks later, I had to give up driving to work and took the subway where I could catch up with a bit more sleep. It was that tiring.

Many young doctors died too in that epidemic. The AIDS virus is not a respiratory contagious virus, they did not die of the retrovirus which the HIV virus is. They died in driving accidents falling asleep while driving.

I gave up driving in those several months. I felt asleep in the car whenever it stopped at the red lights going to work in the morning. It was totally lack of adequate sleep in those few months. (Later months, when more were known about the HIV virus and how it caused diseases and what medication we can use to treat the pneumonia etc, the care was a lot easier). In the current respiratory virus pandemic, I saw a TV picture of a nurse falling asleep at work standing up in China. That created a fatal situation for her. Being tired like that people could catch the virus and could not fight them while 98% of other folks can fight the virus and survive. Why would a lot of the professionals failed to fight the virus? It is merely due to sleep-deprivation.

Studies showed less than 5 hours of sleep makes the immune system useless the next day. The virus fighting cells, the natural killer cells (NK cell, white cells) dropped to 30%. The other white cells like regular lymphocytes and neutrophils greatly decreased too. So are chemicals (cytokines) to co-ordinate the immune reactions. The levels dropped drastically too. That is not a functional immune system.

There is no functional immune system for these poor professionals. Even a cold or flu can be fatal for these individuals.

That is how sleep-deprivation could erode the immune potency. I have experienced the pain of infection with sleep deprivation for a few decades since I have poor dental health (Due to lack of money and knowledge to take care of it growing up, not due to tons of candies). Whenever I did not have enough sleep, toothache came because I have two infected teeth I have to keep for chewing. But the mild infection in these two teeth would hurt if my immune system is a little weak. That happened for a few dozen times in my life. Catching up with the sleep for 3 or 4 days, the toothache would be gone, almost 100%.

Exhaustive exercises erode the potency of the immune system

The times when I did not swim the correct strokes, it was exhaustive. I had many times of sore throat right after those exhaustive exercises that would go away in a few hours. So are the findings from exercise studies. Right after endurance exercise, the immune system becomes weak for 4 to 6 hours. Then the immune system will recover and actually becomes stronger. Moderate exercise would not have the dip in the immune potency.

That explains the observations that marathon runners suffer six times more cold after a race, and swimmers get more colds.

The solution is easy, I stay away from crowds after endurance swimming till my tiredness goes away. But in "steady-states", the swimmers have stronger immune systems and they look younger, so are other athletic people.

How I have gotten rid of the colds for my family members with a supplement. (Either *Echinacea* in the "Zn Lozenge" or *Elderberry* in Sambucol)

The cold virus is called Rhino virus. There is a herbal throat lozenges that can stop the cold/flu from starting or stop an on-going cold in one day or two. That has been a personal clinical experience.

In the online market, I got some throat lozenges for cold called "Zn Lozenges".

Were the throat lozenges useful in the real world? Yes, my wife took it according to the "direction" on the bottle. The "cold" was gone the next day. My son felt the cold coming. He took the Zn Lozenges. The cold never got started. Details can be read in chapter 20.

Do herbal drugs help boost the immune system against earlier cancers?

Maybe, most probably, if the cancer is localized, a restored immune system by the smart lifestyles I mentioned plus avoiding bad foods, most probably could cure early cancers or recurrence. But I am not sure about herbal drugs boosting immunity. There are no evidence-based studies.

Probiotics (good gut bacteria) has the power to control cancer coming back. It makes the immune system stronger (Preliminary studies only)

One study showed taking probiotics (beneficial bacteria) has decreased the incidence (cases) of bladder cancer (focal) recurrence in a population of patients treated for bladder cancer as reported in PDR for Herbal Medicine. In that study, the bladder cancer patients after cancer treatments, were drinking more fermented milk containing probiotics (Yes, I'm drinking fermented goat milk too). They had less recurrence compared to other patients who did not drink fermented milk regularly (fermented milk contains good bacteria for the guts). So better gut-health, better immune system is self-evident. But of course, I think it might help fight the respiratory virus pandemic, though it has not been properly studied through clinical trials.

Vitamins modulate the immune system - Multivitamin –

It is difficult to eat large amount of different foods so we can get enough vitamins and minerals as required. Too many foods eaten will give us obesity. So every guru and every health practitioner recommends taking a multivitamin tablet every day. And I do. In addition, I take regular dose vitamin D every day since it was low in my blood. Low vitamin D is common in about half of the populations especially people who live in the northern latitudes (in the North). Low vitamin D level is said to weaken the immune system. I take additional vitamin C and E, only at regular dose every other days or less. High dose vitamins or herbs or supplements can be dangerous. It is not something I would do lightly. With diabetes, I cannot eat fruits that give a lot of vitamin C. So I take vitamin C. Along with vitamin E, it helps my eye-health.

Does the above smart habits really boost the immune system enough to fight cancer? Yes.

Thanks to the same (old) smart habits, one of my patients did have her carcinoid (means a little cancer) eliminated from her left lung. For months, she worked hard at those habits and lost 3 pounds by 6 months follow up. (This case was described in my other books). She restored her immune potency with the smart life-styling. The smart habits enabled her to shred 3 pounds. Her immune system improved enough to get rid of the "little cancer".

A good immune system is enough to prevent cancer recurrence or even get rid of a "little cancer". So when cancer happens, there probably is some defect in the immune system. Restoring its potency may get rid of a fatal cancer as in a case showed next.

The normal functioning immune system is capable of immune surveillance against cancer cells. Once the surveillance-cells found those cancer cells, they will label the cells and signal the soldier-cells to kill the cancer cells. A dysfunctional immune system with leaky guts cannot do this. Cancer will get the chance to grow, just like my desmoid tumor when I had the irritable bowel syndrome.

Should I believe in "Eat this, and not eat that"? Does it do any good, this new science of avoiding bad foods and eating good foods?

What happened is real. Seeing is believing. Avoiding foods my gut is allergic to I avoided the leaky guts. My immune system was restored like what Molly did. And I avoided the yearly "cold" because my immune system was not misfiring and weak. It was able to recognize the rhinovirus (cold virus) to be a harmful foreign object and destroyed it before it took hold in my nose and throat.

I was at first skeptical of the power of avoiding the wrong foods and eating the right foods, like most health professionals scientifically oriented. This avoiding bad foods and eating good foods eradicating a lot of chronic diseases is almost unimaginable. It sounds like a fairy tale, not a realistic health management. It might just be good little life-style. But little did I knew, I tried it, all the named chronic diseases really got controlled to the degree that I can say they are cured.

So seeing is believing . To my surprise, scientific studies proved the value of these lifestyles of healing the gut boosting the immune system, especially with the gut bacterial studies. I gave it a trial myself and have found it to be true, I got the benefit of curing 33 of my chronic diseases, like disabling arthritis, psoriasis, toothache etc, I cannot help but to believe in the wrong foods and wrong lifestyles were the reasons my immune system failed me in the past and gave me a mild cancer, the desmoid tumor.

Avoiding the wrong foods, avoided hurting the immune system. When the immune system is normal, it is potent. It stopped the yearly cold. It cured the cancer in Molly.

Scientifically, the followings happened:

The foreign objects get into the body through the leaky guts. Leaky guts happened when we eat the wrong foods that we are allergic to, especially gluten. 80% of people are allergic to gluten, though only 5% develops celiac disease like Molly. When there is leaky gut, into the body are billions of foreign objects called antigens. The immune system attacks the antigens everywhere they go, all over the body secreting chemicals to attack them, to no avail because the antigens outnumbered the immune cells and chemicals. The large amount of inflammatory chemicals, the immune chemicals, cause injuries in weakened organs, thus we have either arthritis because the joints are weak, or diarrhea if the guts are weak, or psoriasis if the skin is weak, etc. (They were all weak in me). Thus leaky guts cause all kinds of chronic diseases besides weakening the immune system. The immune system can no longer control cancer cells growing inside us.

Avoiding the wrong allergic inflammatory foods and eating more good foods bring the levels of immune chemicals down, together with good lifestyle like exercises, and good sleeps of six to eight hours, will lower the internal inflammations.

No inflammation in the body leads to no chronic diseases, leads to a stronger immune system. It thus is the basis of the miracle-like changes giving me vibrant skin, black hair, higher energy level, no brain fog, no mood swings, always in good moods, no arthritis and more, since nothing is burning and injuring my body tissues. Some people reported their sex lives become better. Now my immune system works normally. It recognizes the "cold" virus and destroys it. That was how Molly's restored immune system recognized her Kaposi's sarcoma and destroyed it in two months.

How about my taste bud problem with new foods I don't used to like?

Give any foods two weeks. You will find any new foods become tasty. Why? In two weeks, your taste buds cells will all be renewed. The new cells like the new foods. And you will find the new foods delicious.

Where can one find pictures of Molly's Kapos's sarcoma?

In Dr Tom O'Bryn's book, "The Autoimmune Fix", there are nice pictures showing a black patch in Molly's right eye at the right corner. That little patch was the sarcoma, the cancer. In her age group, it usually grows fast and becomes fatal in weeks when this happens in people with weak immunity in which local infection or cancers can spread systemic easily.

In the 1980's, Kaposi's sarcoma was the cause of deaths of thousands of AIDS patients when the disease was first discovered. And there were no good treatments then. (Now there are good treatments. HIV patients' immune systems are kept potent by new medications.

And Kaposi's sarcoma is rare now. Something we all can be thankful for Big Pharma and the researchers to restore the immune systems with strong anti-HIVS drugs. The patients with HIV infections don't die easy anymore). But those bad memories stayed with me, I still remember the horror when I was in my Internal Medicine residence training. The sounds of "777" for resuscitation resonated all over the loud speakers frequently. It was "announcing" that another young AIDS patient was going to die, despite our best efforts of those days trying to understand the disease to save them. Those were the nightmares in the early 1980's for us healthcare workers.

Do herbal supplements enhance the immune potency? (Not sure in the real world, at least in the Western world). There might be exceptions in the professionals who do it all their lives like in China.

Can herbs boost the immune system? I am not sure. One reason one cannot be sure is that the immune system is very complex. Even different cells in the immune system do different jobs, and they help each other or stop each other. We know from laboratory studies some herbs, for example, can increase natural-killer cells in our body. These natural killer cells are capable of killing cancer cells. But small trials on patients did not show benefit.

The Chinese herbs that Chinese herbalists used to help cure cancers are not directed at cancer cells. The Fu Zhen treatment that was reported to increase survival of the pharyngeal cancers patients by 50% in the reported trial in China was aimed at restoring the potency of the immune system. That is what "Fu Zhen" means in Chinese – "to restore to normalcy".

"Treatment" (smart life style) to restore the immune system to normalcy, to achieve the highest potency helps me to get rid of my yearly cold. Just like that.

To restore the immune system to normal to treat chronic diseases has been done successfully on thousands of patients they took care in this country by a new school of physicians practicing Functional Medicine in their offices. These ways of treatments are mostly empirical, that means practically done really, though some of the underlying sciences were shown by small studies. But how many people have been treated that way? They stated that thousands of patients benefited, treated by each Functional Medicine physician. There are thousands of these functional medicine professionals now. So millions of patients must have benefited. There are dozens of books written by these physicians/professionals. The books are listed in the Reference section written by Mark Hyman, MD ; Amy Myers, MD; Sara Gottfried, MD; Jillian Michaels; Michael Mosley, MD; Mihaela A Telecan, DVM, RD; Robynne Chutkan, MD are among the books I read that deals with restoring the immune system with "life style and foods"-The "one smart" move I refer to.

I tried this one smart-life-style-habit of avoiding bad foods, and more than 33 of my chronic diseases are cured or controlled. This included my yearly cold. In this "treatment", some herbs might help. But their use is empirical and not scientific. But the herbs may help as part of the whole life style habits formation.

To Sum Up:

To boost my immunity, it probably will be almost sufficient to remember appropriate amount of *exercise, calorie-restriction and the Mediterranean/Paleo diets*. And some other items would help contribute to a greater immune system like *relieving stress, adequate sleep, eating 80% full and drink a cup of water, and stop,* and *take probiotics* which are the good live bacteria. All of the above are proven methods shown by studies. They will be described in subsequent chapters.

I do not think supplements would be a stronger immune booster than any of the above managements. But in Drs who, all their lives, treat cancer patients with conventional treatment plus herbs, there are exciting reports. One of which showed a 50% better survival. I am referring to the Fu Zhen treatment reported by Peking Cancer Research Center treating pharyngeal cancers.

But such results have not been reported by Western academics because large scale herbal drugs in combination with standard treatment trials have not been done in the West.

With this epidemic of respiratory virus pandemic infection, it is necessary to do immune-system maintenance so it won't be weakened in the fight against the respiratory virus pandemic. Though these still may not be sufficient and avoid exposure is of

utmost importance. Things to do to maintain the immune potency includes but not limited to:

. After strenuous exercise, stay alone for 4 to 6 hours with enough rest. If one's immune potency is very low, more time for recovery.
. Avoid excessive alcohol.
. Practice the health and wellness habits of exercises, calorie-restriction, avoid sugar, avoid overweight, eat plenty of green-leaf vegetable, avoid saturated fats, milk, or gluten containing foods.
. Avoid sleep-deprivation that could have been the cause for the Young doctors, nurses and other health workers dying in the respiratory virus pandemic of (2019) with sleep-deprivation weakened Immune potency.

May God bless the devoted professionals who succumbed, including one of my own co-workers who died falling asleep while driving to work during the height of the onset of the AIDS (HIV) epidemic in the early 1980's.

With HIV infections, I sincerely hope these life-style habits may help to improve the potency of their immune systems (Not including herbal drugs). But of course, only large studies would prove first whether these lifestyles help increase their CD-4 cells etc. And also, such measures are only supplementary to the conventional anti-HIV treatments, and with the treatment professionals' guidance.

Chapter Two - How I man-handled my Erectile Dysfunction (ED)

The fear and the struggle

My control of the erectile dysfunction was a little bit of a struggle. But I "handled it like a man". Thus are the words of the title for this chapter. But in the end, it has been a pleasant surprise.

According to a survey of 3005 people published in the New England Journal of Medicine in 2007, a proud percentage of 53% of the seniors at about 70 years old are still sexually active. I am one of the proud ones. But it takes lots of luck and a lot of doings in tune with most difficult endeavors, though not as hard as climbing Mt Everest.

I have diabetes, the year that erectile dysfunction can set in is at age 60. I was still working as a medical oncologist at that time. When I was not busy, the number 60 would occasionally creep into my mind. So you can imagine how happy I was when I was still able to do it after my 60th birthday.

Endurance exercise boost the testosterone level

What helped me most was swimming 70 laps every other day. Endurance exercise boosts the testosterone level. This male hormone offers great help in sexual drives. And in the back of my mind, the image of the exercise guru Jack LaLanne always reminds me to exercise. Rumor has it he was having sex at age 95, every night. This I would not soon forget. I kept my exercise routine religiously. By the way, exercise besides increasing testosterone level, it saves lives too.

I had a delightful career as a medical oncologist helping cancer patients. I put my heart into work. I believed in the body-power that can also be strengthened to fight cancer. So I dug up all scientific studies that help "cure" cancers by strengthening the body-power to help standard cancer treatments. With these pearls of knowledge, I educated my patients. They almost never had their cancers came back (recurred), and the patients with advanced cancers extended their life span from 10 months to three or five years. These pearls were just condensed from about 500 papers. They are *exercise, 80% calorie diets, relieve stress, avoid sugar, and eat lots of non-starchy vegetables.* These smart life-styling habits did work, and exercise is the most important of them all.

So exercise does save lives too besides saving my sex-life. But let's stick to the topic of ED now.

Retirement brought ED (Don't retire, man)

These smart life-styling habits, led by exercise, saved lives and extend survival. I need to write a book to save more people. So I retired at age 67 to have more time to finish the book "Who is not afraid of Cancers" – One of the main theme was exercise saves lives. After the book was finished, I realize I made a major mistake. The book did not sell that well, so I did not save that many lives. At the same time, my erectile dysfunction (E.D.) started. I guessed I should have stayed at work, and kept busy and kept E.D. away. But it was too late. So at this point, my advice for anyone who is reading and worries about E.D. is simply "Don't retire!" That would do, none more.

First, I checked my medications to make sure no drug side-effect did this to me

The antihistamine Zyrtec could cause ED. I stopped the drug to no effect. So I continued it daily. Later when I use herbs to treat my large prostate, the herb pumpkin seed oil at the dose recommended did cause more ED as it is anti-testosterone. But it was very effective for Benign Prostatic Hypertrophy (BPH-large prostate, not cancer, but it narrows the urine tube and slow down urination). So I used it for a couple of days after the night with intercourse activity and changed to another drugs after two days. More will be said about BPH later in Chapter 3.

Viagra to the rescue

Fortunately, as a retired physician, my finance was OK. So I started the expensive drug Viagra. It did help pretty well. All good life returned. But I remembered quite a few patients had told me Viagra was only effective for about half a year. So I was expecting it to fail in half a year. But it did not fail me in 6 months. Endurance exercise of 70 laps swimming must have helped and kept my testosterone level decent.

But as I got older, the testosterone level would keep declining slowly as a natural phenomenon. After using Viagra at 50 mg daily for one year, I had to increase it to 100 mg daily because at 50 mg daily, penis hardness became a problem. 100 mg daily continued to work.

When the testosterone declines enough as time goes on for the old folks, the Viagra will fail. A somewhat effective treatment would be to see an urologist (The genito-urinary specialist), test for testosterone level. If it is low, then supplement it with medical testosterone by injections or non-injection means. Meta-analysis (analysis of many good studies) showed there is no serious side effects like pulmonary embolism (blood clots in the lungs), or deep vein thrombophlebitis (inflammations and clots) from testosterone treatment. And it does improve ED in a small percentage of people.

I was studying herbal medicine at that time, so I was ready to try herbal supplements if needed, after I studied the side effects and drug interactions of the herbs in PDR for Herbal Medicine.

Never take Viagra or similar drugs when a fatty meal is in the stomach

Fatty foods in the stomach can inactivate Viagra to a certain degree. One time before I took the Viagra, I was hungry and ate about 7 walnuts which are rich in fats. That evening right before the intimacy with my wife, I took Viagra 200 mg (twice the maximum recommended dose plus an extra dose of Citrulline which will be discussed later), I still did not get the absolutely full stiffness of my penis when aroused. It made me worry a bit. But it turned out to be good enough to enjoy the intimacy. So I should avoid fatty meals to eat for the evening of intimacy taking Viagra. So each time I take citrulline and others to help with my ED, and each time I take Viagra, I made sure I took them on empty-stomach, or at least not with a fatty meal in my stomach.

A fortuitous use of one herb helped

After three and a half years, my 100 mg Viagra still kept on working. That was a long time for Viagra to have been working. Was there a higher being looking after me? I wondered. It turned out to be a fortuitously herbal drug I started taking daily. It was *Ginkgo biloba*. It is one of the dangerous herbs listed in books. *Ginkgo biloba* over-dose could be fatal. There are several reports of bleeding complications in the brains and the eyes and irregular heart-beats associated with *Ginkgo biloba*.

How come I am taking the rather dangerous herb *Ginkgo*? There it was in one of the moments of a relaxing walk in the beautiful Northern California. I have a benign tinnitus (ringing in the year) since childhood associated with a mild Meniere's Disease. During that walking along a small river on University of California at Davis campus, I saw a beautiful *Ginkgo biloba* tree swaying in the gentle spring wind. I remembered from my Herbal Medicine learning, it can be used to treat tinnitus, probably because *Ginkgo biloba* increase blood flow to all organs, including the brain (and to the penis, as I would soon find out). So I took two leaves with curiosity to see if it helped my tinnitus. Surely enough, the somewhat loud summer insects humming (the tinnitus sound) became a gentler chorus. Oh, well ... I ordered the herbal supplement on line. At less than 10 cents a day, it was a bargain. Little did I know a bigger bargain was soon to follow! Since then I was taking it 7 days per week at 120 mg daily as recommended in the label of the bottle, though herbs are not supposed to be for long term use.

Why did I want to continue this herbal drug which is potentially dangerous on long term? Dangerous as *Ginkgo* is, its nuts are a favorite food I used to eat as I grew up in Hong Kong. So I was not afraid of it. I just have to be careful not to overdose.

It soon turned out *Ginkgo* has an interesting serendipitous side-effect. Three months after I started the herbal drug, I felt my penis had gained some weight! Yes, that was an honest feeling in the pant. It made sense. *Ginkgo biloba* increases blood flow in the body including the penis.

But studies showed it increase blood flow to the brain especially. So in one study of a group of old folks, *Ginkgo biloba* was given to them. The study was to see if it could improve their brain functions. It failed to show improvement in brain function by evaluation with mental test-scores. But many old folks chose to continue the herb, because it gave them harder penis erections. Well, this piece of the study was not recorded in the PDR for Herbal Medicine. The PDR did not even show it has any aphrodisiac effects at all. But the feeling in my pant that the penis became heavier couldn't be an imagination, because it was very easy to tell. So the aphrodisiac effect was proven to me like a gold-standard trial had been done (Obviously I don't have money for that kind of trial of a few million dollars). And I plan to take it long term. What is there to lose for about 10 cents a day?

Personal evidence that *Gingo biloba* helped ED

One time I ran out of it, and was waiting for the new shipment to come in. I never expected it, but my rather soft penis almost became a disappointment and reminded me I was out of *Ginkgo*. It disappeared a week after I received the new shipment of *Ginkgo* and resumed taking it 7 days per week. The erection became rigid again, and the diameter of the penile shaft was 1.5 millimeter (mm) more with more blood circulated there. I dared never to increase the dose on *Ginkgo biloba* though. It is a dangerous drug. Many people have died from eating too much *Ginkgo* nuts in Asia.

With the help of *Ginkgo biloba*, Viagra 100 mg remained effective. So I could continue living ever happily there after? No, as a medicine man, I know it will not.

A second fortuitous use of another herb helped

Good things always happen in tandem. A second herbal drug joined the gala of herbs dancing with Viagra. That was a popular herb called *Panax ginseng*. It is an adaptogen that can relieve the trauma of stress. Thus it can lower the chronic inflammation inside our body. It is said to increase sexual desire and improve one's physical stamina, especially the ones used in China. This is the red Korean Ginseng from Korea.

But I started taking it for another reason. The reason was to strengthen my immune system so the low grade sarcoma, desmoids tumor won't come back. Many studies have confirmed the immune-boosting effect of *Panax ginseng,* including some studies I read in PDR for Herbal Medicine.

At 20 cents a day, it is worthwhile to take it long term. People have been taking it for thousands of years. It has been safe for them. The only caution is not to take it after noon time. It may cause insomnia then. So I started taking it daily at 500 mg a day. This is a quarter to a half dose. To begin taking herbal drugs, it is good to start at a low dose to see if it is good enough. This is one of the golden rules of using herbs described by herbal gurus. As I said before, I wanted to use herbs to strengthen my immune system for preventing "cancer" from coming back. But it has real sexual uses.

I had a desmoid tumor removed from my left upper jaw 16 years ago. It is not a benign tumor. According to statistics from Memorial Sloan-Kettering Cancer Center, 10% of this low grade sarcoma can kill when it comes back in other sites of the body. I definitely do not want that 10% fatal chance. What Ginseng ought I use? *Korean Red Ginseng* was what I started after researching the internet for a reliable, effective *Ginseng*.

Some say *Ginseng* enhances sexual performance. I was not a believer. I have yet to be surprised.

Accidentally, after taking it for a while, I was given the lucky chance to confirm that *Ginseng* does enhance the sexual potency too. One time I ran out and was waiting for the new shipment. My penile hardness suffered quite a bit. It regained its required hardness when I resumed for a week or so. So with *Ginkgo biloba* and *Panax ginseng* augmenting the Viagra effect, my erectile dysfunction did not return for 4 and a half years. Then as you have guessed, ED threatened to return.

Thanks to a urologist's book

So I turned to a urologist for help, not by asking for more testosterone, but by reading a book by Mark Moyad, MD, MPH (4). Besides being a certified urologist, he is also a herbal medicine guru. Other physicians frequently turn to him for herbal drugs recommendations. From his evidence-based book in the chapter on ED, I selected out L-citrulline, free form, to try to put more blood into my penis when needed? No. But books say it is better to take it daily.

Citrulline almost as good as Viagra (studies)

Citrulline works like Viagra, generating a good amount of nitric oxide to dilate the penis. I hoped to sooth the threat of ED returning. I started with 750 mg of the free form of citrulline. I made sure it is not citrulline maleate which is used for muscle building. It's fine if you want to build muscles with exercise. And again, I started on a low dose even though some studies used a high dose of 9000 mg. I think this high dose may really produce dangerous hypotension.

It certainly helped. No doubt about it. It was easy to make the decision to add this drug, because serious side-effects from it may be hard to conceive and has not been reported. It is one of the nonessential amino acids our body makes. It eventually will turn into nitric oxide that dilates the penile vessels like Viagra and drugs similar to it. It worked wonders for a year.

Now to help Viagra to do the job, I have involved *Ginkgo biloba, Ginseng,* and *citrulline.* The *Gingo biloba* is at a regular dose. Both *Ginseng and Citrulline* are at a quarter-dose. Doing this low dose approach, I will probably avoid the side effects. This eradicated the threat of ED for a full year, making Viagra good for 5 and one-half years.

Then ED threatened to strike again. I again searched for help in Dr Moyad's book (4). I tried *Tongkat Ali,* also called Long Jack. It did not add any effect at this time. There was no surprise. Not everything I added would work at once. Long Jack is supposed to increase the testosterone level. And that takes time to work. So I just continue with Long Jack at the dose indicated in the label. Even though it meant I would be taking four supplements to help Viagra. But two of the supplements are just at a quarter-dose. So I was just taking the strength of about two supplements and a half. But it seemed I was running out of "tricks". But I remembered the idiom, "Where there is a will, there is a way". There was a way, really, indeed!

The greatest help from a study doubling Viagra dose beyond maximum

There is more room for new supplements. There would be a few dozens more available in the market at least. But why didn't I try to increase the dose of the main drug Viagra? So I researched again the studies about doses of Viagra. To my great delight, there was one. In that study, Viagra in its recommended maximum dose (100 mg) was effective in only 45% of the people tested. While doubling the dose to 200 mg, 75% of the people responded favorably. Great, so I doubled the dose of Viagra when I needed it. It was fantastic. It has been the strongest change I have seen in the six years I have been treating myself of ED. I got the feeling conventional medication is way stronger than supplements if used at the right dose, but not overdose. Overdosing may not be safe here too?

The fear of overdose and priapism:

There is always the fear of priapism from overdosing on these aphrodisiacs. Priapism is a persistent and painful erection of the penis (for hours?). It has been reported with the use of aphrodisiacs, though it seemed to happen more often with people who have vascular disease, usually without the use of aphrodisiacs. Priapism is a urological emergency and need to go to ER as soon as possible.

So it's all good. I quite enjoy this good feeling of successfully handling ED, like a man.

Just for academic discussion for now. If with all these treatments, I still fail. What should I do? Two choices: First, see an urologist. Or to increase the dose of citrulline to 150% the dose I am using now, which is at a half dose. Citrulline has been tested in a study against Viagra. It was found to be almost as strong as Viagra. If that is not enough, next is to increase the dose of *Ginseng,* which is also at a quarter-dose only, as long as hypotension does not occur.

Timing is all important

These medications and herbs that increase blood flow to the penis seem to be all short-acting. Their best effects are in the few hours (2 to 5 hours) after taking them. Especially short acting is *Ginkgo biloba.* If I take it in the morning, the effect is very weak by the evening. If I take it in the evening, it helps with penile rigidity a lot. So I take all the herbs in the late afternoon or evening the night of intimacy. That way it would bring out a 100% of the maleness in me.

The herbs and supplements I used and some side effects (not all inclusive):

1. *Ginkgo biloba* – Can make seizure easy to occur. Several case of serious bleeding reported in the brain and in different organs. Stop it two weeks before surgery is necessary. It may cause palpitations and irregular heart-beats. Serious skin reactions have been reported. It can induce seizures in people taking medications for seizures.
2. *Panax ginseng* – It may lower sugar, so caution in use with diabetes. It may excite the heart too much in susceptible people. It may have estrogenic effect, so it should be avoided in people with a history of breast cancers, pregnancy and breast-feeding. Avoid using it after noontime to avoid insomnia. Though it is said to have

estrogenic effect. Its action may be more complicated. Animal studies showed it increases sexual activities. Studies showed it could have increased testosterone level and enhance its action. Sine 5000 years ago in China, it has been used to treat ED, and is still a favorite adaptogen to use.

3. *Tongkat ali* – Very scarce data on safety and side effects and drug-interactions. But old studies on pure stuff worked. Now it is reported some samples from Malaysia were found to be contaminated with mercury and lead. Long-term use may lead to mercury or lead poisoning. Another user-review stated he called the reseller of a Sumatra product who told him the quality nowadays has been compromised. It seemed that there is a supply problem not meeting the demand, and the product may be questionable.

4. Citrulline – It generate nitric oxide like Viagra. Used together may cause dangerous hypotension even though our own body makes the amino acid naturally, but over-taking it may dilate blood vessels too much as to produce hypotension. Another amino acid with similar action is carnitine. But I have not tried it. These amino acids can be readily synthesized, and would not have the supply not meeting the demands problems.

To sum up:

It was a trial and set-back and finally a success journey. Hopefully yours, if you do have the problem, would be a lot smoother. From my ED self-treatment trial experience, I think I found an easy way.

If I were to do it again, I would start Viagra at 50 mg each time or similar drugs under the guidance of my primary care physician. A caution here is to make sure I do not have vascular problems. It is associated with priapism, a prolonged unneeded painful erection, even without the use of Viagra.

As time goes by as we get old, the testosterone level, the male hormone, goes too low. Low testosterone can make Viagra fail. I would discuss with my primary physician to increase the dose to 100 mg, the maximum dose. But keep in mind I can consider a

trial of 200 mg daily. In a study, this does adds 30% more chance of success. Or instead of increasing it to 200 mg per use, I could ask to be referred to a urologist. They can offer many ways to treat ED besides medications, like penile implant, vacuum suction etc, just to name two of the many. The urologist or my primary care physician can boost the testosterone level with injections or skin patches, if mine is low. But testosterone replacement only offers a small chance of success in studies.

There are herbs to increase testosterone levels like what I used. *Ginseng* and *Long Jack* are two examples. But perhaps the strongest way to boost testosterone level is to do endurance exercise and relieving stress, both of which are found to increase testosterone in studies. But unfortunately, endurance exercise is not for everyone. One needs to be cleared by one's own health professional for the endurance exercise. I would do meditation to reduce stress now and then as removing stress would increase testosterone level.

Besides herbs, supplements like Citrulline or carnitine increase nitric oxide which increases blood flow to the penis. It is an amino acid present in our body.

I would add the herbs if I have to, but would do it after try to double the maximal Viagra dose. It would not be that expensive now as it happened to go generic 12/2019.

Last but not the least, if you have not read my "Friendly Reminder" at the beginning of this book, please read it for your safety before consulting your doctor for taking these herbs. And I have to declare what works for me is not a promise it would work for you. Whether it works for you or not would only be clear if you start trying above herbs after consulting your health professional. There are quite a bit of potential dangers from side-effects of the herbs. And side effects may be more serious from individual to individual, including serious allergies. But best wishes.

Chapter Three - A Mixed Drink diagnosed and cured my Benign Prostatic Hypertrophy (BPH)

The beginning of a fairy tale:

The elderly man was seriously ill. He was dying and wanted to die in nature. He left home and went deep into the wilderness in Yellow Mountain where he saw no signs of civilization. There, underneath his feet, was a spring. He was thirsty. He took one drink. He at once felt healthy and strong. Just like that, his fatal illness went away. This was one of the fairy tales I read in grade school in Hong Kong. In story-land, miracles always happen in sacred mountains. I had visited The Grand Canyon, USA, many times. Were there any miracles?

I came to the United States in 1971 to work as a radiation therapy technologist in Memorial Sloan-Kettering Cancer Center in New York City and went to attend a College nearby, one of the many colleges of The City University of New York, after work. Eventually I retired after a whole life working as a medical oncologist/hematologist. I retired in 2002. It was time to visit the sacred mountains in USA. In one of the visits to the Grand Canyon, a miracle happened.

There in a cliff-side steak house on top of the Grand Canyon, right on every table, there was an orange color drink. It was *cactus* and orange juice mixed with a little bit of Vodka. As they say,"When you're in Rome, do as the Romans do". So we ordered the sacred mixed drink to share. It was so yummy. It transformed the gorgeous Grand Canyon valley into a fairyland (Yes, there was quite a bit of Vodka in the drink). In fairyland, miracles happen all the time.

We bought a bottle of the *cactus* extract home. Bought a big bottle of Vodka, and mixed the same drink almost every day. All of a sudden, without warning, my urinary-stream became wide-open. It was so forceful that it hit the toilet bowl with a drumming sound, so loud it was close to a distant thunder. The sound was so different than the very silent urinary sound for the last 10 to 15 years. I thought the old slow urinary stream was a matter of aging. The urine flow rate had been slow. Now it was fast and strong. It was a miracle. It happened after visiting the sacred Grand Canyon. After drinking enough of the *cactus* mixed drink for a while, my wife did look a lot younger too and looking more beautiful. It was just part of the miracle, nothing to boast about.

I got Benign Prostatic Hypertrophy (BPH-enlarged prostate) and didn't realize it. Only after it was shrunk by *cactus pear* and the urinary stream opened up then did I realize I got BPH. But that was not the end of the world, of course. I did quite enjoy the mixed drink.

My primary physician confirmed I had a soft lump on my prostate with normal test of prostate specific antigen (PSA). It was a benign prostatic hypertrophy, an enlarged prostate but not cancer. But it compressed the urinary tube (urethra) and slowed the urinary stream.

How did the *cactus pear* shrink my enlarged prostate?

The *cactus pear* had shrunk my prostate, by getting rid of the old cells that did not want to disappear from my prostate like it was supposed to. Now the *cactus pear* made the old cells break down their cellular inside, wrapped them up in small membranous particles and just disintegrated away to be reused by growing cells. The whole process is called apoptosis. Apoptosis is a Greek word depicting the beautiful falling leaves. *Cactus* causing apoptosis was shown in laboratory studies. But when I stopped taking it for a few days, the old cells accumulated again and narrowed down my urethra (the tube which urine passes) again. The urinary stream would become smaller and weaker. So I continued eating *cactus* fruit and later switched to using *cactus pear* supplements.

The *cactus pear* has been used by elderly men for hundreds of years in the country side of Sicily, Italy, for urinary problems. *Cactus pear* for BPH is not as well-known as a few other herbs. But it is getting more and more attention. Now you can order it as a supplement of *cactus* extract in a capsule. One capsule of 500 mg a day, drive my BPH away. It is less than 10 cents a day and can be ordered online. And I did not suffer a common fear side–effect of conventional BPH treatments. The side-effect is impotence. Many of my patients told me they stopped the conventional drugs for BPH because of this side-effect. Blessed be to this little *cactus pear* capsule, now I don't have to hunt for *cactus pear* fruits in the supermarket like a madman anymore. The *cactus* fruits were rather hard to find.

Financial fairy-tale happened

I use Nopal by Solaray for my *cactus* supplement. It is controlling my BPH very well. At the cost of 30 dollars per year, this is a financial fairy tale. It is a fairy tale if you realize it takes me less than a penny a day. I believe herbal medications have a place in American healthcare. It certainly will lower the cost of healthcare if it is widely accepted in USA.

USA is the only country where herbal medicine is not used alongside modern medicine. In Europe, doctors can prescribe herbal treatments when appropriate. Their healthcare cost is 50% of USA. But their health statistics is superior.

By the year 2040, our healthcare cost is projected to be equal to our National Tax Income. That is to say, the total amount of "money" produced for the USA government is just enough to cover healthcare. I think widely and wisely using medical herbs will lower the healthcare cost. It is obvious to see. If we don't do it, we are like an ostrich hiding its head deep in the sand when danger approaches.

My understanding of some herbs on the market for treating Benign Prostatic Hypertrophy (BPH)

The chemical in plants called beta-sitosterol is the main ingredient that can shrink the enlarged prostate. If the herb contains beta-sitosterol, it should work. If it doesn't work and the herb is said to contain beta-sitosterol, there may be quality problem of the herb. The effect should appear in a few hours or so with *cactus pear* in my experience.

All herbal drugs have some side effects. They should be studied well so you could know about the herb and its *side-effects* and *drug interactions*, then discuss taking it with a knowledgeable health professional before start taking them.

Even the seemingly harmless *cactus pear* that is consumed daily in large quantities in some countries as food has side effects. It can lower your sugar. I never felt hypoglycemia (low sugar) with it because my blood sugar is slightly high due to diabetes.

Next I'll just bring up some popular herbs and mention some information that I think would be interesting to you.

1. *Saw Palmetto*: This is the most popular herb for BPH in USA. I

would never use it for one thing. I have read a case it caused impotence in one of the herbal guru's book. It does contain beta-sitosterol if it's the real stuff and the right part of the plant used.

But various studies on it do not persistently produce a positive result. It gave me the impression of being 50:50 effective. In fact, two well run studies by the US government showed *Saw palmetto* to be not effective. The Urologist-Herbalist guru Dr Mark Moyad called it "worthless" in his book "The Supplement Handbook".

2. ***Pumpkin* seed oil:** I am taking the *pumpkin* seed oil cold press capsules at 1000 mg per day, two days per week. I used it because it may shrink the prostate size by reducing prostate tissue. This effect was described as due to anti-androgenic effect. So I only use it 2 days a week or so for fear of ED. The rest of the time, I take *cactus pear* supplement at 500 mg a day. Whenever I used the *cactus* supplement, the urinary stream became strong always the same day.

Pumpkin seed oil rarely has side effects. It may upset the stomach. It could lower the interest in sex probably because of its anti-male hormone effect. But botanical plants have very complex chemical ingredients, not like pharmaceutical drugs having one and only one effect (but they are strong). *Pumpkin* seed oil is conductive to hair growth. That is an androgenic effect like male hormones. The *pumpkin* seed oil has a molecular conformation (shape) similar to 5-HT (5-hydroxytestosteone, the more active form of testosterone). It could combine with 5-HT by fitting to the molecular structure of 5-HT and cancel its effect out in the prostate, but it may foster hair growth like testosterone for hair follicles, that is my speculation. My hair looks better than before when I was taking pumpkin seed oil.

3. ***Cactus pear*** - After cactus pear controlled my symptoms of BPH, I tried to look up why it works that way. But most literature only says it is consumed in Latin countries as food. It may control diabetes, obesity or cholesterol problem. But there are no scientific studies I could find to prove that at all. So how does it make urinary stream strong again?

More searches showed studies revealing the reason of *Cactus* treating BPH is by apoptosis. The old prostate cells fail to go away and build up a large prostate. *Cactus pear* as described earlier in this chapter can make old prostate cells go away by stimulating apoptosis.

Some of its side effects include mild diarrhea, nausea, bloating and headache. Like all medications, it is contraindicated in pregnancy and breast-feeding. It may lower sugar in diabetic people and cause hypoglycemia (low sugar problem). Besides, it may make adjusting glucose (sugar) level difficult during surgery.

4. *African Pygeum* - This supplement has been given high mark in various herbal literatures I read. The regular dose is about 100 mg daily. Side effects include nausea and upset stomach. But the list of side effects here is not all encompassing. I have not tried this myself. I cannot find it in the PDR for Herbal Medicine for more side effects.

     I mention this herb because the studies are frequently showing it is effective. It is reflected by its increasing demand, such that some African countries encourage investment for large scale cultivation. It's a popular herb for BPH in Europe.

5. **Stinging Nettle** - It's approved by Commission-E (German official authority on Herbs etc) for kidney and bladder stone problem, infections of the urinary tract, and rheumatism per PDR for Herbal Medicine. But various herbal literatures describe it for BPH also.

     A prospective observational study of 2080 subjects reported in PDR for Herbal Medicine, when combined with *Saw Palmetto* for 12 weeks increased urinary flow and decreased night urination times by about 50%. Only side effects reported was gastrointestinal upset in 12 people, 6 of them discontinued the trial. This is not a randomized placebo controlled study, so called gold standard trial. But if it is approved by official for rheumatism, it is anti-inflammatory, good for the control of chronic diseases. So I mention it as well just to point out *Cactus pear*, with its lack of scientific studies, was described to help with knee pain in folk message forum. So *cactus pear* could be anti-inflammatory too. My arthritis problem was at one time near disabling. Now it is almost all gone (When I kept up my exercise - more on that in the chapter on arthritis - chapter 5).

To sum up-(And present some relevant discussions about lowering healthcare money).

     To sum this chapter up is just brief. Accidentally, I

discovered *cactus pear* can shrink my enlarged prostate and return the strong urinary stream. For 10 years, it keeps on working. I will continue with it as it is effective. It also poses very little threat of side effects. Why? In Latin countries, it is consumed in large quantities, and without serious side effects. Besides, there are *cactus* farms supplying large quantities of it. Unlike *African Pygeum*, the *Pygeum* trees are not that fast growing. Therefore the supply has been dwindling. Then may be in the future, whether you are getting the real herb would become a problem.

    <u>Soul searching discussions centers on money</u>. Pharmaceutical drugs are expensive NOT because people are greedy. Its research work in the laboratory before discovery is expensive. It often is the one chosen out of thousands tested in the lab. Once the drug is discovered to be good, its tests on human subjects involved many distinguished hospital systems and well trained scientists, physicians, and statisticians. That is a lot of money. Then the cost of advertisements is huge too.

    In short, the money involved to produce this single drug is astronomical. That's why the price of the new drug is so high. By comparison, the "birth" of a folk remedy is entirely free. Hundreds of years and millions of people used it, if it is effective, so it is accepted by users as good, like most herbs we see on the market today. Persistent effectiveness is almost like a golden study. And most can be ordered online. The herb's being around is almost like a natural selection by users. It won't exist for hundreds or thousands of years if it is not effective. That's the golden test of time.

    So now for one penny a day, I am controlling my enlarged prostate, enjoying a good quality of life with easy peeing. At this cost, this aspect of the healthcare cost in treating BPH is cheap. This is good news in a country that may run out of money for healthcare. Believe me or not, this country is USA.

    In Europe, there is a government appointed committee for approving herbal medications called Commission-E in Germany. And doctors can prescribe herbal drugs when indicated.

    Their healthcare cost is 50% of USA, yet the health statistics are superior. So is it time now we should have an American

Commission-E? And start teaching useful herbs in US medical schools?

Why is this necessary? It is due to the escalating healthcare cost. It is estimated that by the year 2040, which is 20 years away, the healthcare cost will be equal to USA's total taxation. It just makes sense to lower healthcare cost now.

Chapter Four - How I got to look alarmingly Young - Personal anti-aging secretes

Exercise keeps us looking young, the first thing:

How come I and my wife looked like in our 50's while we both are actually older than 70 years old? It is due to four smart lifestyle habits. Earlier in our younger times, exercise was the only habit that was enough to keep us look young. We were not as old then. Now we need to employ all the smart habits to look healthy and young. I will describe them one by one in this chapter. There are four smart habits totally that together, keep us looking young. If I deviate from one of those habits, as I found out in real life. I will look older in a short span of time like in days.

But first, I want to reflect on an incident that looking young can get you in trouble.

Just how young did me and my wife look by swimming every other day? Very young, when we attended our high school re-unions in San Francisco, there we have a few dozen high school classmates who are still alive. We were so young-looking, we could double as their children. (No offense, classmates, folks. People would say anything when they write books. Remember the Chinese saying: Scholars BS a lot). That's how young we look. Of course, most of them looked their age of 70 years old or more, though a few of them looked young too.

A pair of young looking crooks:

Now imagine we looked like a couple in their 40's or 50's, yet our drivers' licenses say we were born more than 70 years ago. And it happened in a bank. We went there to set up a new account as we moved to Florida from New York for the winter. We requested to transfer more than ten thousand dollar from a bank in New York. The hot Florida sun tanned us dark and looking more sinister, and I guessed being a Chinese American couple didn't help either. That was very suspicious. Did we try to swindle some poor old folks in New York out of their life-savings? Very possible.

The bank lady was startled when she saw our dates of birth not fitting our young looking faces. She went away from the office with our driver's licenses to check "something". The process of opening an account took three hours. Imagine you could do that in five minutes in another bank Capital One as they advertised themselves to be. Our bank account did take three hours to open (To be fair, it was a special account). No doubt there was a lot of time spent on security-checking on us suspicious looking Chinese couple is my guess. Oh, well, whatever, we got the account opened. We are retired. Time is not that precious anymore.

But growing old and looking old is not pleasant. You want the four smart life-style habits, right? Ok, right now.

So the first smart life-styling habit for anti-aging is EXERCISE

My exercise is lap swimming every other day. It took me three years to make my free style swimming smooth so I can swim 70 laps without over-exertion.

Not only do I look young, I feel good with the endorphin level increased with exercise. The other books I've written fully explored the benefit of exercise in cancer control and the scientific evidences were presented as well. It's worthwhile to spend time in one of the three books. (They are sold at cost and available online).

The latest proof that exercise is anti-aging is in the genes

In one major study, the Nurse's Health Study, the nurses that do a lot of exercise (like running 3 hours per week) have a longer tail (telomere) in their gene complex. Since the older humans become, the shorter the tail. The longer tails in the genes undeniably means they are younger biologically. To me exercise increase my endorphins, causing a higher level of male hormone of testosterone is good enough for me. But I like a longer tail in my DNA-complex too.

Ok, you don't trust in science. You are looking for things happening in real life about being forever young. Here is one finding from the book of a health guru. One of his friends called Frank is an avid swimmer in his middle age. Once Frank was in a luxury hotel attending two conferences on the same day, the two different conferences are in different halls for different societies. One meeting was for swimmers like him. The other meeting was for insurance agents like himself. As he left the swimming conference and entered the insurance meeting, he realized he had just left a group of fit and trim young-looking middle age folks like him and entered into a hall full of middle age persons with prominent bellies and looked decades older. This is the real world. There have been many times I remembered some fat belly males glancing at my belly with a long look and a pair of self-pity sad eyes, even though I am not that slim.

Lower your chronic inflammation inside your body, your outside will look good and young

The next one in line to make you look young and fit is lower your internal inflammation inside your body. Then your outside would look good. This chronic inflammation can be shown by doing blood tests for inflammation chemicals which are higher than normal. When these chemical levels are higher, people have more chronic diseases. Aging itself is like a chronic disease. So we know inflammation is related to a higher chance of chronic diseases. These so called chronic diseases are every disease in the book, like diabetes, hypertension, metabolic syndrome, obesity, asthma, arthritis, heart attack, stroke, skin blemishes and yes, cancers too. And aging is considered one chronic disease. That is, no internal inflammation means no aging look.

You don't necessarily have to do blood test for chronic inflammations. When inflammation inside is high, though, you can tell by the appearance of a lot of signs and symptoms due to chronic diseases. Your skin would look older. Eating the wrong foods, my skin is no longer shinny, my face shows more wrinkles, my diarrhea due to sensitive gut system comes back, acnes appear in my face again, I would be feeling depressed, anxious, or not sleeping well etc. These are signs I feels when I'm down and low with high internal inflammation. For me, the signs of a higher level of chronic inflammation are acnes and diarrhea and looking older. The skin system and the gastrointestinal system are my weak points in the body when inflammation attacks. Spider-web lines appear, psoriasis is becoming obvious, along with a slight limp of arthritis to complete an old-looking picture.

Lowering inflammation is the 2nd key to look young. It can even lower PSA.

One friend I knew for 40 years from the community swimming pool was found to have an elevated PSA. Work-up was negative for prostate cancer. And he had no signs of a big prostate. He is not a smoker also. Smoking is known to raise PSA. So he has no reason for an elevated PSA. But it does happen, making you worry about an oncoming prostate cancer. The PSA story will be described in Chapter 27. I just want to say here, as his PSA went down, he looked much younger because he shredded 7 lbs as the inflammation went down with diet I mentioned to him.

I studied a lot about foods and inflammation. There was a study showing eating a lot of pomegranate, tumeric, broccoli, and green leaf-vegetables lowered the PSA. That was all he had to do, eating more green-leaf vegetables.

Anti-inflammatory foods will probably cure your chronic diseases or control them, and making you looked very young

The foods my friend took and his PSA went down are called Good Foods. Please read Chapter 39 for more details. My friend's PSA went down not only because he ate the red, yellow and green vegetables mentioned above. But also he was living the healthy life habits-because he also lost almost 7 pounds in six months. This naturally happens when you eat the good foods, tune up the immune system, and heal your guts. You don't have to try to lose the weight.

Good foods can really make you look young as I will show in the next few paragraphs.

Did I believe in the power of foods on our very health, including looking young?

I once happened to watch a television episode of Dr, Mark Hyman debating a famous surgeon (Not Dr Oz) about the merits of food affecting our health. The surgeon proclaimed loudly, "Eat these, and don't eat that (for health). This is not medicine!" followed by loud applause and mocking looks from the audiences.

With similar college and medical school education programs as the surgeon, I should have applauded his speech too. Because in medical schools in America, the priority for nutrition topics are low compared with millions of medicine related topics. That is a shame. After I studied the effects of diets on health in the past few years after retirement, I realized these topics should be taught more extensively and be included in different medical board examinations Why? Are you sure?

Yes I am sure. Eating a lot of the anti-inflammatory foods, my irritable bowel syndrome is gone. My mood swings which were mild, but my wife insisted it was horrible, is gone. My skin looked silky, not loose, dry, scaly and with fishtail lines. In fact, I got more than 30 chronic diseases cured or controlled by, "Eat these, and don't eat those".

What happened if I am not careful and eat whatever foods I like?

Ah, that did happen last spring when I went back to New York, after more than 6 months in Florida. For two weeks, we dined out almost daily in Chinese restaurants with their tasty greasy foods, Italian restaurants with their rich Italian bread, Thai restaurant for the sweet Thai tea; and fried foods, plenty of fast foods and refined carbohydrates, processed foods. These are all bad foods but tasty. I am just human. It was heaven!

Trans fat increases chronic inflammation, causing chronic diseases

Its not that I didn't know restaurants are using trans fats for cooking and they are largely exempt from the ban since 2013 by FDA. Trans fat taste good, it makes food last long. It is cheap. It is banned from use by large scale manufacturers because studies showed it clog arteries, causes stroke, heart attack, type 2 diabetes, and increases the risk of colon cancer. Restaurants are largely exempted.

But in me, trans fats caused chronic diseases. Before I knew, my diarrhea came back due to my irritable bowels. My skin no longer looked silky. It was covered with wrinkles. My hair was greyer than black and my mood swing came back. All the above changes were due to increased inflammation inside my body. As you recall, inflammation causes all diseases known. Different people get different set of the combinations of the chronic diseases.

Trans fats causes chronic diseases and brings aging

How do we know trans fats increase inflammation? The Nurses Health Study showed it. For nurses who consumed trans fats, their blood test for inflammation, CRP was 70% higher. The CRP is a very sluggish test. When it goes up, the increase in inflammation is real bad.

I had to stop "eating whatever I liked" and back to eating only "good foods". It did not take long. In another two weeks after eating anti-inflammatory foods, just like magic, my skin regained its silkiness, the hair was almost all black, frequent diarrhea stopped, my black psoriatic patch on my left knee faded. Fairy tales as these sounds like, but it is a true miraculous change in real life. If you don't believe it, saying it is fairy tale. Give it a two to four weeks' trial, you may see the fairy tale come true for you. *That is why I believe in "eat these, and don't eat those". It works.*

The 3rd item to make you look young - Reduce your stress:

Reducing stress is easily said than done, some would think. But, no, it is easy if one takes it methodically. Exercise is the best for me to reduce stress. So I started my crawl style swimming 3 years ago, style change from a life-long breast-stroke swimmer. Why, free style swimming is easier and it can do endurance swimming. I was really slowly crawling in the beginning. It took forever to get to the other end of the pool. And it was not pretty, though I got it done. But methodically, I remembered the teachings of free style swimming from books and videos. After a few dozen corrections over the last three years, I finally can swim smoothly and do 70 laps (if I want to) without struggling. You just have to be persistent. Don't give up or give in.

Other means to reduce my stress is to do the things I like only if it is good for me. So a lot of fishing, sailing, take care of grand children, and listening to music on my earphones. But most important technique that really helps relieve stress is meditation. I learned it from studying books in high school. Meditation works magic for stress release. Now if I need stress release, I close my eyes, direct all my attention only to deep breathing. I try to feel how the air smoothly flow through my nostrils, how my abdominal muscles rise and fall with each deep breaths, how the rest of my body muscles are all relaxed. In my mind, it helps the relaxation by counting the numerals 1, 2, 3 etc, counting each number multiple times. I can refresh myself in 5 to 15 minutes, or even a few seconds. I would recommend it to anyone. Go read books or learn it from instructors. It will calm and enrich your life.

People who do mediation often have a different brain activity pattern, more brain in the positive and calm areas by brain scans in studies.

In scientific studies, a less stressed person has lower inflammatory chemicals in their blood. In the long run, they will have less heart attacks, strokes or cancers. These points have been born out in studies, not an imagination. So go take deep breaths with your eyes closed, body relaxes with nothing in your mind but the awareness of your breathing movements, or do yoga, Tai Ji, pray, ride a stationary bike, loop jumping provided you are in shape. I can't jump loop much. But philosophically, what do I think is the best way to release the stress every day? They are exercise and mediation whenever I need.

The best way to release stress is to have no want, a good philosophy

Advertisements are teaching us to want this, want that, day in and day out. But remember, enough is as good as gold. I think that is the biggest thing that relaxes me, that is, to have no want. This no-want mentality definitely has a lot to with the Confucius teaching I underwent in high school in Hong Kong. So the mentality of righteousness, no greediness, observant of all the rules and taboos, do a lot of good for me. "To have no want" is taoism but it is also imbedded in Confucian teachings.

I wonder whether this teaching of "have no want" should be included in elementary education so children won't be totally led with hooks to their noses to chase materialism relentlessly. Some can argue this "motive of want" is going to increase productivity of goods for the country. But in actuality, this is a heavy mental burden. There is always something more that you want. It never ends and it torments.

The real problem is that "want" has no limit. It will only drive everybody to live on their credit cards. That should not be part of the real life. To have no want, but work and get what you need, is the right attitude in children education. They will grow up happier without a heavy mental burden of "endless wants". In other words, they will have less stress, and less inflammation, less diabetes, less asthma, less heart attacks, less strokes and less cancers. This is the real benefit of "no want".

Now there is something to release stress that everybody

agrees on.

Last but not the least in reducing stress is simply sleep soundly daily. Sleep six to eight hours a day. Do not watch too much TV too late. Sleep deprivation is the number one reason in America to bring big time stress. Stress induces inflammation. Inflammation makes you looked your age or older most probably. Exercise is the best way to bring me deep sweet sleeps.

Another "last but not the least", this one is the easiest.

There is not going to be big talks for the 4th secret to acquire looking young. The last one item to make you look really young is sun-tan lotions, creams, ointments, or sprays. That is when you have silky skin, no fishtail lines, and baby skin on your face. Definitely, a young face is the key to looking young.

It takes a lot to make the face look young surgically. And it is expensive. But here is something cheap, the sun-tan lotion on the face before exposure to the sun, every day. So remember to put on your sun-tan lotion on the face, hands or any part of the body that is exposed to the sun. With global warming, the sun no longer burns, it scorches. This started in 1993. That was the first time I felt burning on my skin under the sun in the summer in New York. The New York summer sun never burned my skin as long as I could remember since 1971.

So from that day on now and then, I put on sun-tan lotion before I went out in the summer, but not always. But finally, I firmly remembered to put on sun-tan lotion every single day before I went out in the sun. I did that after I saw a badly scorched face in the boathouses area in Sausalito, California. The skin of the face of that sailor looked like coarse sandpaper. I would rather look at the face of a cadaver in the anatomy lab. Since then, I put on sun-tan lotion each and every time before I go outdoors. This is the most important part in the fight of anti-aging. If the skin on the face doesn't look young, a person doesn't looked young.

So to sum up:

First thing first, don't look too young for your age when you are in a bank transferring a large sum of money. Then to look young, first remember sun-tan lotion. Then do appropriate amount of exercise. Eight to ten hours of slow walking per week, 2 to 3

hours slow running, 2 hours fast running, 2 to 3 hours swimming or stationary bike riding per week etc. Four key things to do to remain young: Exercise as mentioned, release stress, lower your inflammation, apply sun-tan lotion. Lowering chronic inflammation is the most important to achieve good health and looked young. This can be done by avoiding bad food and eating good foods. It will be discussed in Chapter 39.

But other smart living habits are very important too, like enough sleeping, social supports, amusements, regular meal times, larger breakfast, small dinners and other healthy living habits.

It's not difficult to look and feel young. The habits mentioned in this chapter are real and "proven" by studies. Be persistent and learn to practice them and you will be healthy and looked young.

Chapter Five - How I gained back my Freedom of Movement and healed my disabling Joints

(*Exercise to the rescue but needed stem cells to leave my bone marrow, and the control of inflammation*)

I busted my own joints. But luck was on my side. The impossible combination of 3 to 4 fortuitous events saved the joints. Otherwise I certainly would have been disabled by now. The saving grace was thought to be due *only* to the mechanical grinding from exercises. That was what I thought at first. But more brand new sciences I learned revealed that a lot more fortuitous events had been involved. It needed an endurance exercise to make the bone marrow to release enough stem cells to settle in the diseased joints. The stem cells change into cartilage cells, bone cells and other joint cells. So the patch-up repair could be done, yet those patch-up repaired joints were good enough for gentle functioning only and could not be abused.

Motion is lotion: Exercise, the first fortuitous event

So far there were four fortuitous events. Fist was my routine exercise that moved the disease-joints gently while swimming. This gently grinded the joints smooth. Injured joints tend to repair themselves with forming new bone-tissues. But it is done in disarray (reactive bone formations), like building bone spurs between grinding surfaces that ended up stopping joint movements because it is painful to rotate the joints with bone spurs in-between. Exercises seem to be able to grind away such abnormally-formed bones between joints. That was the experience on my own joints.

Second event that help mend my joints: Endurance exercise "harvesting" stem cells naturally from bone marrow to circulation

Second was the endurance exercise which stimulates the bone marrow to release more stem cells from the bone marrow into the circulation. When I swim, I usually swim 70 laps in a 25-meters long pool. That makes the distance I swim of 70 laps to be a mile. So that there would be enough stem cells released from the bone marrow and circulate, and to home in the diseased joints as the **third fortuitous event**. Stem cells are primordial cells that can model themselves into any structures as required, like patching on bones, cartilages, or ligaments. But these repaired parts are patch-up works rather than as good as the original parts of the joints. But they are good enough for regular use without pain or problems interfering with movements.

 The last fortuitous event was perhaps the most important. It is to create a low inflammatory condition in the body. Only under low to no internal inflammation conditions, then the repair work of the joints could go on.

 These four steps happened without me knowing it when my joints were repaired as I exercised. Neither did I know this complicated sciences of joint repaired. It just happened. But to know these sciences is to do joint-repairs naturally with a good chance of success.

Fourth lucky event needed to mend my joints: Reduce inflammation

 An expert in the "battle-field" of Stem cell Regeneration Therapy of the joints (mainly) pitched in one more important information. Without controlling the inflammation, the joints could not have been repaired even given tons of stem cells as are given in their clinics. I had suspected that controlling inflammation was necessary. Then it was confirmed. And it was necessary and essential. All these fortuitous events, unplanned and unasked for, happened to me just like that and healed my joints: 1. Exercise to smooth out the joints. 2. Endurance exercise to release more stem cells from the bone marrow. 3. Stem cells could access the injured joints to change into different tissues of the joints. 4. Reducing inflammation in my body so joint repair can start.

I just kept on working on my good life-style, and good things happened to my joints.

 I wanted to strengthen my immune system, and I started lowering the inflammation by avoiding bad foods and eating good foods, that ended up helping joint repairs. How lucky could that be? This made me believe in a higher being, and believe in extreme luck in destiny. I am grateful and extremely humbled at the same time. But how did all these needed steps for joint repair happen? And just what happened that I got my joints busted? Can it be described in videos of daily life so it is easy to learn? Yes, of course. So let me start from the beginning.

Over-use caused joint injury. Arthritis showed up a year later as a result of the injury a year before

Now back to the beginning, how did I hurt my joints? That was twenty years before my retirement. It all began with the purchase of an old sailboat. It was a sturdy 28 ft. sailboat called Erickson 28+. It was cheap. It cost less than an ordinary used car. But it needed a lot of physical work to rejuvenate the boat. We loved the boat. The boat could survive a storm if driven the right way (I think I never had the chance to try yet, though my wife may disagree).

So for the weekends in the following two months, my wife and I were in the boat yard, grinding, sanding, cleaning, painting, waxing and varnishing. My joints were overtaxed with that huge amount of physical work. But at the time, there was no pain, though the joints were injured and I didn't feel it, because I was too excited to have the chance to go sailing on our sturdy sailboat.

Right shoulder "frozen"

In the years following the injury, my body's repair-process built a lot of abnormal little bones protruding between the joints. They are called bone spurs. Eventually, they severely limited my joint movements. I could not reach back with my right hand. The pain would stop me. Nor could I raise my arm above my right shoulder. My right knee was hurting too. I walked with a limb and could not do much physical work with my right hand. The disability was obvious.

When I was working in California near San Francisco, an orthopedic surgeon friend noticed my disability in movements while I was limping a little in the hospital. The surgeon offered to operate on my right shoulder in two weeks.

The weekend before the operation, I went sailing in San Francisco Bay. It is a tough place to sail in San Francisco Bay. It is said that "if you can sail in the Bay, you can sail anywhere (in the world)". It was somewhat true. The wind is always shifty and violent. One time my boat got turned around by a sudden gust of swirling wind 360 degrees in seconds. I didn't brink my eyes, because they remained wide open for a couple of minutes. The boat wasn't scared. It just sailed on.

Thus this is San Francisco Bay. Some old salts (very experienced sailors) proclaim there is a whole fleet of small sailboats on the bottom of the bay sailing under water, back and forth, carried in and out by the currents of the daily tides, till eternity.

Backhand grab to a life-line suddenly freed my right shoulder from being frozen

This one time, all of a sudden, the boat tilted. I was falling onto the deck. The life lines were behind me. My right hand reached back and grabbed the line to stop my fall. Doing that, I broke the bone spurs that limited my right hand from reaching back. Just like that, I avoided surgery to my right shoulder! That was quite unceremonious. So grinding out the bone spurs saved my day, and I thought that physical grinding was all it took to heal a joint. It turned out it actually need more lucky steps, I just didn't know it at that time. That sailing incidence was the first of several fortuitous events that saved my joints.

Overhead reaching gradually freed my right hand from inability to reach up, without me realizing it

But there was still the problem of raising my arm above my right shoulder. That needed another fortuitous event. Without knowing it, gradually, my right hand reaching further and further up above my right shoulder in learning the free-style swimming. Finally after a year or so, I was able to raise my arm above the right shoulder and pointing it straight ahead of me. It was physical grinding again in the free-style swimming that did it. That took a whole year when I switched to free style swimming from my life-long swimming style, the breast stroke.

A terribly long time had passed before I finally realized I broke all the bone spurs limiting my upward movement of the right shoulder. That was how fortuitous it was.

As for the right knee, I knew right away when the pain was gone. It was the result of one of the warm up exercise I acquired from the swimming books. That warm up exercise for the right knee was just a lot of moving my right knees back and forth with the help of my right hand. All my weight was on the left leg which was slightly bent in this warm up exercise. One warm-up exercise of my right knee for thirty times, I noticed right away my right knee pain was gone when I was walking to the pool to swim from the warm up area!

So it did seem that physical grinding was all I needed.

Motion is lotion. Is it enough?

So I thought. It was all due to the grinding of the joints that had done the healing. I could not have been more wrong. First, after the grinding job, there is a need for some stem cells to come to the joints, to mature into bone and cartilage or ligament, whatever was injured.

So this time I did not realize, I need a lot of stem cells, not just a few stem cells that usually is continuously released by the bone marrow. Stem cells are immature cells residing mainly inside the bone in hollow spaces of the bones called bone marrows.

Stem cells only leave the bone marrow and go into circulation one at a time or so, being constrained by a net-like structure called the bone-marrow-to-blood barrier. So the second thing I did not realize, I got to get a lot of stem cells to go out of my bone marrow and be circulated to my injured joints without the junks in the joints hindering the access.

Bone marrow releasing stem cells to the rescue

So the second fortuitous event was to get a lot of stem cells to be released by the bone marrow to go to the injured joints after the grinding job. The grinding job was the first fortuitous event. Now I need a lot of stem cells.

New science showed doing endurance exercise, a lot of stem cells will come out of the bone marrow, into the general circulation. Endurance exercise indeed when I always swam in the pool for 2 to 3 hours. The exercises itself mechanically circulate away the "junk" from the injured joints out to the circulation to be taken away, so the stem-cells can gain access.

No lowering the body's inflammation, no repair would happen

Another major fortuitous event was lowering the chronic inflammation in my body. Inflammation means my immune system is attacking foreign objects and secreting inflammatory chemicals to burn the foreign bodies dead. Those chemicals are causing the chronic inflammation. The inflammatory molecules of the immune system will create wounds faster than you can repair them if the body has chronic inflammation. So you need to cool down the immune system to cool down the inflammation.

I purposely ate a lot of green-leaf vegetables because I knew it was healthy to do so. I didn't know at that time it was anti-inflammatory to eat a lot of non-starchy vegetables. That I learned later after I retired. So these fortuitous events all combined to give me my usable joints back. How lucky could I have been?

The mended joints are good just for gentle use

Are these repaired joints as good as those formed when I was in my mother's womb? No, no way. I could get these joints hurt real easy. For example, it would hurt if I ignored the warm up exercise in which my arms swinging in circles for 30 times each arm. Without these warm-ups, I would feel the pain when swimming. So the joints are not perfect. It needed maintenance work of all the three major fortuitous events: 1. Joint-Grinding from warm up exercise and during exercises, and to be continued through daily activities. 2. Lots of stem cells from endurance exercise. 3. anti-inflammatory foods. The need to keep eating good foods that are anti-inflammatory is obvious. If I ate too many bad, inflammatory foods like sugary foods, or too much greasy foods in the restaurants using trans fats for cooking, I will feel joint-pains few hours later in my wrists, no exception.

How can I be sure that stem cells can repair joints? After all, this is fore-front medicine that has not been proven. (Though a lot of clinics are doing joint repairs by infusing stem cells – not FDA approved). I felt it is a true useful treatment when I saw an x-ray picture of a shot-up lower back (lumbar spine physiologically fractured in many places). It became a perfect spine after stem cell treatment. These radiographs (X-rays, and CT's) were shown in a conference given by a Chiropractic in Florida, a clinical group doing Stem Cell Regeneration Therapy (mainly for joints?).

And I heard, "All the stem cells given won't work if the inflammation is not controlled...and ...you cannot run on concrete roads any more". This I guessed was a statement from the experience of seeing and treating thousands of patients in more than 20 years of practice. One has to lower the inflammation in the body so the stem cells would work. And the joints after treatment are not as strong as the original joints, as I understood.

To sum up -

from my personal experience and my understanding from a conference in stem cell therapy of the joints: (Please bear in mind these are not results of "gold studies" and such therapy is not FDA approved).

Personally, I think joint repairs involved grinding in warming up exercises, plenty of stem cells to leave the bone marrow to repair the joints can be achieved by endurance exercises (This one is the result of scientific studies)**. But most important of all, there is a need for lowering the inflammation by eating good foods (see Chapter 39). Eating good anti-inflammatory foods lowering the body's chronic inflammation was observed in a lot of studies.**

And the repaired joints need maintenance exercises with warm-ups, and the patched up joints are just good enough for functioning without pain and cannot be physically abused. These are only my personal experience, not results of studies.

Chapter Six - How a Shingles was cured at the rash stage with topical *Tea Tree* oil (cost - less than a dollar. Never have pain again from shingles!)

The basics of shingles

Let's review something almost everybody knows. 80% to 90% of the children were infected by the shingle virus when young. Most of the infections may appear like having a mild cold. But the shingle virus called V*aricella zoster* becomes dormant and hide in our nerve tissues. When our immunity is weak, Shingle can happen. Shingles is an infection mainly in the skin by the re-activated herpes virus that resides in our nerve ends when our immune system is strong. When the immune system is weak, they reactivate themselves and infect the skin. In times of stress, it can happen too. (Stress or the fact of getting old weakens our immune system). Half of the elderly can come down with shingles. In half of the people, as the shingles (rashes) on the skin heals, it is followed by a painful nerve pain sometimes described as "hell-fire". If we kill the virus at the rash stage, no "hell-fire" will happen.

Shingles first appear as a rash on the skin. The rash distributes in a belt fashion draping around the body, but involving only half the body stopping sharply at the middle. So physician seeing that half-body only, curving distribution, would be able to diagnose shingles. The shingles rash is followed by blisters. When blisters rupture, it oozes. That is the stage that is contagious by direct contact with the fluid. Then the ulcerations healed and "hell-fire" follows. That brings misery and burning pain that no one would forget.

Herpes zoster rash on the skin

Not a good thing to have. But my wife unfortunately was chosen by her destiny to have it.

It was one of those hot and humid weeks in the summer in New York. But we were enjoying a cool breeze in a rented cottage by the lakeside in the Pocono Mountains in Pennsylvania with our extended family of eight people for our annual gathering. In that cool morning in our bedroom, my wife showed me three crops of rash in a belt like fashion. It was only itchy a little bit. The rash is clearly a shingle rash to me. This retired old doc (Me) have seen many such rashes of herpes zoster (shingles). We were hours away from emergency rooms. But by that time, I have learned quite a bit of herbal medicine on my own. I brought some medications for the trip. *The Tea tree oil fits the bill.* It is broad spectrum antiviral, anti-herpes, antibacterial, and also anti-fungal. I also had a stronger essential oil, the *Oregano oil.* I originally brought it along for mosquito bites and "no-see-um" flies bites. *Oregano* for flies, and the *Tea Tree* oil for mosquitoes.

One bottle of these essential oils is extracted from about sixty pounds of the herbs. The word essential means "the essence". It is highly concentrated. Some of them are pretty caustic. But not *Tea tree oil.* This *Tea tree* is a small tree, not the same trees for tea.

Tea Tree oil was also specifically found to be anti-herpes in studies.

Tea Tree oil cured the zoster rash in one single day

So I used a cotton tip, soaked up some *Tea tree* oil. Spread it on the whole belt of skin (dermatome) including the two crops of rash. The good skin along the belt was covered too as the virus may already be present underneath the belt of skin. I left one crop of rash free of *Tea tree* oil, leaving it for *Oregano oil.* The thinking was good. In case of failure with *Tea tree* oil, I would need a more potent oil---the *Oregano oil* to put on the third crop of rash. Boy Oh Boy, as soon as the *Oregano* oil touched the rash, it was found to be a mis-step. That was a mistake of not realizing the rash skin was not intact skin anymore. It was so strong, it created the "Hell Fire" on the third crop of the rash. It hurts me even now to think about the pain when my wife was suffering from the *Oregano oil.* I hurriedly soaked up the *Oregano oil* from that particular crop of rash. But it took quite a few minutes before the hellfire pain was gone. Yet it is better than a few weeks of post herpetic pain with similar hell-fire like pain.

In the evening, we spread *Tea tree oil* again on the rash. In just half a day, the fresh-looking rash in the morning was already withering. We had taken photos in the morning when the rashes looked fresh. By the evening, the photo showed the rashes withering. It worked. In three days, the rash was about gone, though the scars took about a month to disappear. But my wife never had blisters, skin ruptures, ugly crusts and the "Hell-fire" post herpetic pain.

If every patient can detect the rash, has the chance to use *Tea Tree* oil to kill it. Then millions of patients in the world every year will be spared of the "Hell-fire" pain. Wouldn't it be great? **I think this treatment needs to be explored and if found effective, be adapted into conventional treatment**. (Unless a new equally cheap anti-viral can do the same job, I wish).

Why does the *Tea Tree* oil makes killing virus look so easy?

Plants grow up from the soil which is full of microorganisms of bacteria, viruses, and funguses. Yet plants still flourish generation after generations. They either can resist the microorganisms or have weapons against all the bacteria, virus, and fungus. And most essential oils can get rid of most of the micro-organisms. Humans have discovered their antibacterial and anti-viral properties for a long time. In fact, *Tea Tree* oil was the hospital antiseptic before the age of the antibiotics in the world. Now they are still being used as such in the whole world outside of USA, especially in the developing countries.

I have conveniently cured a shingles (Herpes zoster) at the rash stage just like that, and my wife was spared of the 50% chance of a serious pain of shingles that can last for weeks or months.

Case confirmed by a certified dermatologist

Half a year later, my wife visited a certified dermatologist who is expert in skin disease in medicine. The dermatologist looked at the photos and confirmed the case was Zoster and it was cured by the *Tea tree* oil. The amount of oil we used was less than twenty cents. This is really cost-effective. I am glad I had confident in the antiviral and anti-herpes property of *Tea tree* oil. So we avoided using oral Acyclovir which only lessens the disease course a little if taken early enough. Any medication that fights DNA to get its effect is not my favorite. Also the vaccinations I really don't like. They are far from a 100%. But honestly I realize these advices are for myself only. It is not sound conventional medical advice.

For shingles at the head and neck area, I would not try anything other than conventional medical antiviral treatment. Zoster at the head and neck area has been known to cause blindness or even death, rarely, even when treated with conventional anti-viral treatment.

But that is the proper treatment.

One should not be thinking about Tea Tree oil intravenously. It could certainly be fatal.

Health professionals with hearts unite to eliminate "Hell-fire" from the face of earth! (Note: Not a Christian war)

How can this be done? Buy a $10 bottle of Tea Tree oil to put in the primary care office and Emergency Rooms and use it for shingles. But it may need the government or TV services to run advertisements showing the pictures of early zoster rash distributions so patients know to go for treatments early. Lastly, I hope the ultraconservative medicine men and women are receptive to this suggestion without doing clinical trials. It's hard to do randomized studies as there is no telling any enrollees will develop shingles and no one can induce shingles for the sake of studies (There is no safe way of inducing herpes re-activation). Readers who read this book would most probably develop a strong immune system and probably will never develop shingles.

To sum up

For shingles (Herpes zoster) that appears outside the head and neck areas, I would use *Tea Tree* oil on myself anytime. It is safe to use (only) topically. But a few cc taken internally can be fatal.

To me, it kills the virus, and the disease disappears when the rash heals, and then normal skin comes. There. No blisters, no crusting, no post-herpetic pain. Any of the signs of shingles just mentioned above, the antiviral drug acyclovir fails to get rid of. It just lessens those symptoms. And I used less than a dollar's worth of *Tea Tree* oil.

Chapter Seven - How my Allergy was cured

In this chapter, I have two allergies that were cured. One pollen allergy the other one was year-round allergy (Probably to house dust). An episode of pollen allergy was "cured" in three minutes with a roadside plant in the year 2011. It was only a temporary cure as this happened back in the old days before I learned about the Paleo-like Mediterranean diet. The diets are anti-inflammatory. It could improve and calm down my immune status so allergies or "asthma" can be cured "permanently" along with a myriad of chronic diseases. This sounds like magic. But the healings were backed by new scientific discoveries and thousands of patients cured with the Paleo-like/Mediterranean diets. So I decided to give it a try. And it eventually cured both of my allergies so silently that I did not even notice.

I didn't realize my year-round allergy was gone

I started the anti- inflammatory diet early in the summer of 2018. About 30 chronic diseases of mine were cured in a month, as if it was done by magic. Yet I didn't realize my year-round allergy was one of the cured chronic diseases. I continued my daily half dose of Zyrtec. Till one year later, I said to myself, "Smart lifestyle habits cured a lot of my chronic diseases, may be the year-round allergy is gone also". I stopped my Zyrtec to see if the symptoms of the year round allergy are still around. Sure enough, I had no more allergy symptoms even without the Zyrtec. No more runny-nose, no brain fogs, no stuffy nose. Prior to this, I had been taking Zyrtec for more than 10 years for my allergy which I never bother to find out the cause. (I had the clinical feeling it was dust allergy).

I cured an episode of my Hay Fever in three minutes with a shrub by the roadside. (Talking about instant medical effects of the herbs)

About 15 years ago, I was in Northern California, working as a medical oncologist. I lived near San Francisco. The weather was like spring year-round. Flowers bloom all over the place with luxuriant trees mostly year-round. They spread the fragrance and the pollens in large amounts. My life-long allergies required anti-histamines daily. But it did not help if the tree and flower pollens were plentiful. I had to add steroid nasal spray whenever necessary.

It was in one of those lovely spring days. I was walking with my wife along a trail by the bank of a small river in the University of California at Davis. We were walking in a fantastic world of flowers and trees from all over the world. They were transplanted from all over the world and cultivated by the horticultural faculty and students. We were an hour away from our car with a full box of tissues in the car. I only grabbed seven of them with me. My eyes were tearing. My nose was running with a continuous dripping of fluids. Six tissues were gone. Only one tissue left. It was a dire emergency.

Right at that moment, I glanced at the hillside. Some plant attracted my attention. There was a lovely green plant with needle-shaped leaves. It was a *California Ephedra*. It is a great anti-allergy tree. It was my "life-saver" for sure. I picked 7 tips of the leaves, chewed and swallowed it down in a hurry.

I kept on walking, my nose kept on running. I used up my last tissue. I was starting to lose hope and prepared to pull my T-shirt off for drying my nose. Right at that moment, my eyes dried up, my nose stopped dripping. It dried up too. Then I could breathe again. That took 3 long minutes. So this was my hay fever stopped in three minutes. Glory be to the *California ephedra.*

Glory be to the herb*s, no!* Right at that moment, my heart had a round of forceful palpitations for two seconds. It pounded my chest wall. Then I remembered this plant was known to cause fatal irregular rhythms of the heart if overdosing on it. It might have been better if I just took three tips of the leaves. Ten or twenty tips of the leaves probably would have been enough to stop my heart and kill me. In 2004, *Ephedra* was banned in USA. It is banned all over the world. So never overdose yourself on herbs, especially the dangerous herbs.

So I stopped the vicious attack by hay fever in 3 minutes with *Ephedra* plant. But it was dangerous and banned. What did I plan to use?

I was taking Zyrtec, it was then the least sedating antihistamine on the market. Later, friends told me Claritin was more non-sedating. I tried it. It was just a bit less sedating than Zyrtec to me. But I was used to Zyrtec, so I continued my daily Zyrtec at half dose.

By then, I was pretty knowledgeable with herbs. One of the

anti-allergy herbs has no sedation. It has been used since the times of the ancient Romans and Greeks. This herb, *Butterbur*, is very popular in Europe now. I was about to try it with the precaution to buy the PA-free *butterbur* supplement. PA stands for pyrrolizidine alkaloid that is present in this herb *butterbur*. Pyrrolidzidine is toxic to the liver and even can cause liver cancer if taking it for a longtime. I'll have to make sure what I buy is PA free. Besides this one, there are several others equally good without sedation. *Stinging nettle* is equally good. *St John's Wort may be effective.* Or I can just take quercetin for a week before the allergy season begins. That works too in studies. They are all good herbs or supplement hat have multiple great beneficial effects in the body besides treating allergy.

Allergy-free without any drugs! Thanks to the diets

But drug-free is always better. As I said before, right at that time in mid-summer of 2018, I had already practiced the all-important, life-changing smart life-styling of eating Paleo-like diet (see Chapter 39) for about a year. A lot of my chronic diseases disappeared with that diet, including allergies. Since I discontinued the daily anti-histamine, my mind became clearer, my dry-eyes relieved. Thanks to the anti-inflammation diets which let me be allergy-free while drug-free.

The life-changing habits are just knowledgeable healthy living habits of choosing to avoid bad foods and eat good foods, just the one smart lifestyle. What are all these smart lifestyles?.

Smart life-style habits: (That together got rid of all my chronic diseases, allergies included: It strengthens the immune system and calms it down to be strong). (Please see Chapter one for more details):

.**Exercise:** Long known to enhance the immune system. It boosts immune system by various means. It was all from studies. The underlying sciences were elaborated in my other books sold at cost, available on line.

But there is a caution with exercises. With strenuous exercises, there are a few hours after exercises that the immune system is temporarily weakened. One should stay away from sick people that have infectious diseases during those 4 to 6 hours.

.**Eat till 80% full:** It takes 20 minutes for an already full stomach to tell the brain to stop eating. If you eat till full. You eat too much and would gain weight. Gaining weight in studies was shown to weaken the immune system. So eat till 80% full and drink a cup of liquid so the stomach is distended to give the feeling of 100% full.

.Relieve stress: Stress increase inflammation in our body. Blood test will show their presence. Inflammation weakens the immune system. Adequate sound sleep (6 to 8 hours or more) is a strong stress buster.

.No sugar - Americans eat the most calories from sugar, from a Tuft University study. The sugar is in the form of high fructose corn syrup (HFCS) it is in all processed foods. Why is it bad? HFCS is sugar. Sugar is inflammatory. It is also the only fuel for cancer cells.

.Keep the same weight (i.e. don't gain weight). Weight gain is gaining in fats. Fat cells make inflammatory chemicals. Inflammation weakens the immune system while being hyperactive to cause allergies.

. Eat good foods, avoid bad foods. The good foods are lowering inflammation in our bodies. Bad foods cause inflammation.

. Sleep at least six to eight hours a day. Inadequate sleep is very inflammatory. It has weakened immunity for the young doctors and nurses who over-worked, not had enough sleep and died of the mild Respiratory virus pandemic infections. (They could easily die from the winter cold in those temporary immune-compromised states).

The above were the old smart lifestyles which work together to lower inflammation and calm down the immune system, but still it did not calm down my immune system enough because of my irritable bowel syndrome. It needs one additional smart move to get rid of the allergies and my other chronic diseases. The one smart move is just to avoid eating bad foods.

I was at first suspicious of the power of avoiding the wrong foods and eating the right foods is powerful enough to affect my health. But as more scientific studies proved its value, and I tried that myself and witnessed the benefits, I am a firm believer. With 33 chronic diseases of mine, including my yearlong allergy controlled, by avoiding inflammatory foods and eating anti-inflammatory foods, I cannot help but to believe. Scientifically, it let the followings happen.

1. Eating good foods mend my leaky guts.
2. The now tight gut walls results in no foreign objects absorbed from the colon to be circulating inside the blood. Without billions of foreign objects in the circulation, the immune system will not be exhausted and become over-active and thus be dysfunctional.
3. Then there will be no more uncontrolled immune soldiers attacking everything insight, becomes hyperactive, hyper-responsive that a harmless thing, say, like pollen, would initiate immune response which is allergic reactions.

The one smart lifestyle of avoiding bad foods and eating good foods finally brings the levels of immune chemicals down enough. It thus is the basis of the miracle-like changes of no allergies, vibrant skin, black hair, higher energy level, no brain fog, no mood swings (in good moods), no arthritis etc as described in the chapters in Part One. Some people reported their sex lives become better.

To sum up – (What got rid of my allergies?)

Whao! With so many good lifestyle habits, which is the one directly responsible for controlling my allergies? The answer is perhaps all of them but the lowering of the uncontrolled immune hyperactivity by avoiding bad foods maybe the most important. Now no foreign bodies gets in my systems, there is no immune war. The immune system has been calmed down and controlled, and not over-reactive which is allergy. So it is mainly the one smart-move I did of "Avoiding the wrong foods, eating good foods" that has done it finally. I can see newspaper articles telling some kind of foods affecting allergies all the time. A study showed children with asthma had fewer asthma attacks in the group of children that consumed more green-leaf vegetables. They ate more good foods! They had less asthma attacks. The kids would be smarter too.

Please believe in anti-inflammatory foods for your kids. Your kids would most probably be more clear-minded and have no mood swings. They maybe more calm to receive good advices. Thus they may achieve a lot more in their future.

Chapter Eight - How I got rid of acnes and made my skin a more vibrant younger skin.

How bad was my skin?

I found some suspicious-looking black spots on my skin in my right leg thirteen years ago. So I went to see a dermatologist in the medical center where I worked as a medical oncologist in Northern California. In the leisure time, I spent a lot of time under the sun. So watching out for skin cancer and checked those skin lesions early was a wise decision. Check skin cancer early can mean the difference between life and death. What I did not expect was my skin was so ugly that it could scare a dermatologist.

When the dermatologist was lifting my trousers to see my right leg, he dropped the pant-sleeve suddenly as if he had seen the skin of a devil. My skin was dry, scaly, full of spider-web lines and had some flakes sticking to the socks. I guessed he did not expect a respectable oncologist, his colleague, should have such despicable skin. I was embarrassed. So I uttered meekly," I used skin cream everyday". He took a real deep breath. Calming himself down, he told me to use ointment instead. So I have been using ointment from then on. And I discovered ointment is a lot thicker than cream.

In the end, what mattered was that the spots on my skin were not melanoma, a potentially bad cancer. I was Ok with my ugly skin. I thought to me self, "this was not my fault, my mom gave this skin to me". Born pre-matured, there got to be something bad. I never could have imagined, my skin could look silky and smooth too, same as the dermatologist would be expecting.

The skin on my face was another story. At age 63, it looked young and Ok. I put suntan-lotion on my face every day for fear of getting malignant melanoma, a bad skin cancer. For the skin in the legs, it still had to wait to get better. The skin ointment did not change the skin in my lower legs a lot. It remained dry with spider-web lines and skin flakes, just less with the use of ointments. It remained in that despicable condition for years. It's OK, it's hidden by trousers.

Paleo-like/ Mediterranean diet (see chapter 39) transformed the look of my skin in the leg and hands.

But despicable skin can become vibrant skin in someone who keeps on learning new sciences. Joy to the world, this happened near Christmas time of 2018. What happened? "Eat these. And don't eat those" again? You guessed right! How and Why?

Why not? Thousands of patients treated by the Functional Medicine physicians, mainly healing the guts with smart life-style-changes worked well for the patients. After the internal inflammation is lowered, their skins become vibrant with acnes gone. That is mainly empirical results they observed. I tried it for myself like that. My life-long acnes were gone and my skin looked a lot better. With this 70-some-years-old skin, I cannot declare it vibrant. But maybe it's close.

How does lowering inflammation get rid of the acnes?

Modern studies do support this skin transformation. There is finding that chronic inflammation makes the hair follicles "sticky". This would slow down the oil (sebum) from transiting the hair follicle-tunnel to lubricate and protect the skin. If it is severe, the sebum can clog the hair follicles, and the bacteria Cutibacterium acnes (formerly called Propionibacterium acnes) will grow in the sebum resulting in acnes. So lower chronic inflammation indeed will let the oil go out and lubricate and protect the skin, making it looked vibrant. No clogged hair follicles means no acnes.

Did I comply with the diets a 100%?

A 100%? No, I am just a human.

80% of the time, I avoided wheat (gluten) and wheat products like bread and cakes. But I avoided foods like sweet cookies 99% of the time. 100% of the time, avoided milk, thanks to my lactose allergies. 50% of the time, I avoided cheese, in the past. But from now on, I will try o avoid cheeses 100% of the time which I learned recently they pose cancer risks. (It will be elaborated in Chapter 39 about how bad cheese can be). Almost 100% of the time, I avoided processed foods and sugars.

Nonetheless, my skin was transformed. No obvious spider web lines.

To sum up:

Just like magic, my life-long acnes that took me a lot of face-washing and scrubbing with soap under running-water from the faucet, every morning. Now it was suddenly gone. I don't have to scrub 3 to 7 tiny acnes off my right temple area every morning no more. (I left the large ones alone, if it were there).

While I followed the smart life habits that dwarfed cancers (see Chapter one), the acnes still occurred. My skin looked rather old then. I still had my irritable bowel to take care.

But after I also tried "Avoid Bad Foods, Eat Good Foods " for a couple of months, my acnes went away and my skin looked very decent. Life is good after my immune system stops attacking the hair follicles. Now there are no more clogged hair-follicles to cause acnes. And sebum (oil) could go through the hair follicles onto the skin, protects the skin and makes it look waxy and shinny, and yes, looked younger.

Chapter Nine - How my Diarrhea from Irritable Bowel Syndrome disappeared

A huge 10 to 20% of the population has this Irritable Bowel Syndrome (IBS). In me, it mainly manifest as diarrhea. If you are one of them, you have my sympathy for the misery. Hopefully this chapter will help you "sign out" of the embarrassment and eliminate the inconvenience of making sure there is a toilet somewhere in your daily life.

Was my IBS a problem?

In the past, I paid very little attention to this problem, because the bathrooms were just a few steps away in the hospitals, in the office, and at home. And a busy physician was not supposed to go anywhere else that may not have toilets anyway. Not too inconvenient, and my diarrhea was painless.

Actually, it might have been good for me to have those frequent quiet times (Sitting quietly on the toilet) so I could get out of the hectic life for a few minutes often. No wonder my character was so mellow. Ha! I have only discovered it now. I must admit it was a good way to release the stress of a busy life as a medical oncologist. Anyway, all my life, while in the bathroom, I was only called by my pager twice while tending to my IBS. That was in more than 40 years. And answering the phone sitting on the toilet-bowl was not that difficult. And if IBS got out of hands, 0.5 mg of loperamide usually made the feeling go away and the diarrhea stop. I never needed a full pill for fear of the side effect of constipation.

What caused my IBS?

IBS may have multiple causes and nobody really knows for sure. Traditionally it was believed to be related to the brain-gut connection, hyper-motility, and small intestine bacterial overgrowth (SBO) etc. All those were studied to be possible causes. Now people concentrate their studies on food sensitivity and the gut bacteria. There have been plenty of studies too. But for me, the wrong food is the cause each time. And the real important thing is how to get rid of the diarrhea and the felling of constant urgency (to defecate). I studied the problems and came out with practical solutions---avoidance of bad foods, for me, it is mainly greasy foods of trans fats in restaurants and fresh fruits, and of course, milk and cheese. That sounds simple.

I found out I have milk intolerance. And milk or dairy products will cause diarrhea in me soon after consuming them. So I do as everyone else would. I avoided milk, dairy products. Also a lot of foods have to be avoided too like a lot of fresh fruits, greasy foods, coffee, tea, and tomatoes and some more.

There was still the gut hypersensitivity (Urgency)

Foods avoidance worked. I stopped getting diarrhea frequently. But my gut hypersensitivity was still there, the annoying feeling of urgency was still there. So there must be more to my IBS. It was not simply food allergy.

There was more. May be my guts were not healthy. Yes, there was inflammation in my colon discovered by colonoscopy. So it was back to square one. The internal inflammation caused the feeling of constant urgency, because it causes inflammation in my gut walls too. So I turned my attention to the hip things: Gut health and gut bacteria and Paleo-like/Mediterranean diets are the hip things. They lower the internal inflammation.

Unlike other hip trends, though, this one of lowering the inflammation is showing its power on controlling every chronic disease like stroke, heart attack, arthritis, asthma, allergies, and cancer. I think this trend is not going to disappear like all others before it. This trend of gut health and diets for the gut bacteria is going to stay.

It probably will make it into medical school textbooks in the future, because it is effective in improving the general health, physical and mental. And it will help control all chronic diseases, IBS being the one at focus now. Because I tried lowering my internal inflammation and the feeling of constant urgency of IBS is gone, along with all the chronic diseases discussed in this book.

Now let us get back to IBS. Food sensitivity is one real thing responsible for my diarrhea. That may not mean it is also responsible for the colon inflammation. This morning, I ate half a tangerine. It did not occur to me I cannot tolerate a lot of fresh fruits. Now I am having loose stools. But the sense of urgency is not there. So it is the colonic inflammation seen in the colonoscopy that really caused the sensation of urgency, not the foods.

Now the urgency is gone. I just cannot wait to see whether my next colonoscopy would detective a normal colon without inflammation or not. I really look forward to the next colonoscopy showing normal colon surface without inflammations.

The thing that got rid of my urgency is the Paleo/Mediterranean diet. The main point in the Paleo diet is to avoid foods brought out by agricultural revolution. These food items can easily be committed to memory by remembering what is commonly eaten for breakfast by especially kids. Remember what foods are in a bowl of cereal: Wheat, milk and sugar. These foods were not present in the Paleolithic period of Old Stone Age. Our genes may not have the tools to digest them. The gene-set evolved and might have become more or less fixed millions of years ago.

Agricultural revolution only was started 10 thousand years ago. It brought a whole lot of new foods from agriculture and animal husbandry. Now we have milk from another species of animal for us to drink daily (which is not healthy-allergic proteins in milk from another species). Because now you got a cow so tamed that she would stay put as the farmer squeezes milk out into a big pale. Imagine you asked a husky wild cow in the Old Stone Age to let the caveman do the same. No caveman would be that stupid anyway.

So milk was what the cavemen/women did not have besides wheat, and sugar. Milk, wheat and sugar, my old Paleo genes just do not know how to digest them, and my gut got hurt each time I eat those stuff. My guts are sensitive to those foods.

So the one smart move I made was the same old thing –Avoid bad foods and eat good foods.

What kind of foods I eat to avoid IBS?

Now my daily food is very Paleo-like and Mediterranen-like. Half a plate of non-starchy vegetables cooked with plenty of olive or coconut oils which are good fats that we need. The other half plate is good meats low in saturated fat, like chicken, fish, chick peas, and grass-fed beef. My breakfast is mainly good proteins and non-starchy vegetables and eggs. No sugar, milk, cheese, gluten or dairy products nor salt. I allow myself one egg per day. My cholesterol is not high. And anyway, in 2015, the US Dietary Guideline Advisory Committee

finally declared, "lowering cholesterol did not lower the cardiovascular risk", after hundreds of studies showed this fact in the years past. But "be careful with saturated fat" is still advised by every authority.
Good fats lower internal inflammation. So 20% good fats of or so of the total calories is encouraged nowadays, so is a larger proportions of proteins in meals being the normal now.

To Sum up:

A big part of healing my Irritable Bowel Syndrome is due to restoration of my gut health by eating Paleo-like diet and Mediterranean like diet, mainly avoiding foods not present in the Paleolithic Times of Old Stone Age. The reason is that our digestive genes were set by the time of Old Stone Age, more than a million years ago. The main foods to be avoided are wheat and wheat products, milk and milk products, sugar and salt. These foods appeared almost a million years later than our old genes had completed their evolution.

Personally, there are a lot of foods I have to avoid for now: Milk and milk products, wheat and wheat products, sugar, salt, coffee, tea, tomatoes, some fresh fruits, greasy foods, trans fats, processed foods, high fructose corn syrup. Yet I still have plenty of foods to choose from.

Life is a lot easier when I don't have to look for a toilet because of diarrhea from the irritable bowel syndrome. And then my brain-fog is gone, my mood is a lot more mellow, my joints are pain-free to say just a few.

Chapter Ten - How I understand it's still possible for me to have Heart Attacks though my Cholesterol is not high

The pendulum keeps on swinging back and forth. Time keeps on ticking. It ticks away old theories and installs new ones. Low fat low cholesterol diet to decrease heart attack is out. Inflammation as the cause of stroke and heart attack is in.

Low fat, high carbohydrate diet caused 60% people to be over-weight and increased in fatty liver disease

About 50 years ago, low fat diet was the recommendation of all health authorities and organizations. Two generations of Americans eat by such diets. But excess (starchy) carbohydrates in this diet got turned into fat by the liver, promoting weight gain. Now 60% of Americans are overweight, 30% are obese. Why high (starchy) carbohydrate diet caused obesity and increasing fatty liver disease?

Those high carbohydrates diets, especially the high fructose corn syrup (HFCS), or simply labeled as "fructose" get absorbed from blood readily. They got carried to the liver faster than other sugars, along blood circulation. Other sugars travel through the slow lymphatic channels. Right in the liver, the liver cells turn HFCS into fat for storage. There is no choice for the liver except to turn HFCS into fat, (Unlike other sugars with choices of turning into fat, triglycerides or be spent as energy). HFCS-derived fats flooded the liver environment. There comes the epidemic increase of fatty liver disease and obesity. HFCS in processed foods is the major source of calories Americans consume, according to a study by Tuft University. These HFCS-derived fats can constrict and hurt our arteries giving rise to heart attacks and strokes.

So you can see the reason why the low fat diets actually increased fats for us, and raised heart attack and stroke risks. But does cholesterol cause heart attacks and strokes?

Lowering cholesterol did not lower heart attacks and strokes

Finally, in 2015, the US Dietary Guideline Advisory Committee clearly declared, "lowering cholesterol does not lower the rate of cardiovascular events". All other health organizations agreed in the face of hundreds of studies saying so. Therefore, low fat diet is out, though saturated fat is still considered bad.

Chronic inflammation is responsible for heart attacks and strokes

About twenty years ago, studies started to show chronic inflammation caused plaques to form in our blood vessels. It also causes plaque-ruptures which are responsible for heart attacks and strokes. But then one can asks, if inflammation causes heart attacks and strokes, lowering inflammation should decrease heart attacks.

But for 20 years, it was hard to prove that until recently. It was shown in the CANTOS study, a gold-standard study, showing that decreased inflammation led to decreased second heart attack by 15%. In the CANTOS study, a single inflammatory switch, one of the interleukins, was silenced by an expensive monoclonal antibody made in the laboratory. Can eating good food match that effect? Evidence from studies showed it is so, and much more effective.

There is a switch at the nucleus of a cell called NFKB. Trans fats can turn it on, so is a dense piece of white bread. Once it is turned on, NFKB can make 150 inflammatory molecules. So if we avoid eating trans fats (in processed foods), and avoid lots of white breads, we won't generate all those inflammatory molecules. To lower inflammation, bad foods avoidance probably will be stronger than a single monoclonal antibody.

Though I am sure that monoclonal antibody is turning off a very important switch called interleukin 1-beta. But avoiding bad foods saves us from all those inflammatory switches being turned on in the first place. No need to worry turning them off, because dozens of pathways won't be turned on if we avoid the bad foods.

One example of lowering inflammation, lowers heart attacks and strokes

That is why even when a patient is having dangerous level of inflammation like in Rhematoid Arthritis (RA) patients, with disabling joints, with pending heart attacks, can still become normal people just by avoiding bad foods, eating good foods. RA is a bad disease that inflammation can attack any organ of the body due to a dysfunctional immune system attacking everywhere. (See chapter 1 for details)When the blood vessels of the heart are attacked by internal inflammation, they cause heart attack accounting for 50% of the deaths at young age in RA patients.

How inflammation cause heart attacks, not the cholesterol

studies also showed the higher the inflammation level, the easier it is for the plaque to rupture. Once the plaque ruptures, it exposed denuded wall of the blood vessels. Clots will form there. If the clotting is big enough to obstruct the heart vessel, cutting off oxygen to the heart muscles that depend on that particular blood vessel, that area of the muscle die and that is a heart attack.

These plaques-formation and plaques-rupture has nothing to do with cholesterol. Inflammation starts it and finishes it all. Cholesterol is just one of the stuff to be used to build up the plaque, regardless of whether the cholesterol level is high or normal or even low. It doesn't matter.

That is why if one's cholesterol is normal, heart attack can still happen, especially if one has positive family history of heart attacks. In fact, fully 50% of heart attacks occur in people with normal cholesterol levels. My cholesterol levels are normal, but that does not say I won't get a heart attack, especially if my inflammation in the blood is high.

Chronic inflammation happens if we don't have good gut-health as described in Chapter 1, 9 and others. How does chronic inflammation affect the blood vessels? We can see the explanations in patients with rheumatoid arthritis (RA). It has a heightened inflammation level as a result of immune system dysfunction.

The result is chronic inflammation in the blood attacking everything, including the blood vessel walls. The leaky gut wall is the reason for inflammation in RA also. In hundreds of patients with such diseases treated for gut health with Functional Medicine physicians. The patients resolved their rheumatoid arthritis (RA) just by avoiding bad foods. In the Chapter on spontaneous healing (Chapter 41), there will be cases of RA patients healed by lowering the inflammation with foods and smart lifestyle- habits.

RA patients commonly have severe inflammation of the blood vessels and have higher incidence of heart attacks which are responsible for 50% of the premature deaths in RA patients. The inflammation in their blood vessels is called vasculitis which is very hard to treat with conventional medicine. The treatment for RA is worse than the disease with lots of disabling side effects. But treating gut health by avoiding bad foods often do it, and is easy. As long as the bad foods are made known, then it is just a simple matter of avoiding it to avoid heart attacks and strokes and disabling arthritis.

When the blood vessels of RA patients are so severely inflamed, the vessels can become weak, thickened, and narrowed. The inflammation in my blood when I got the desmoid tumor (with a weakened immune system) probably was not so high to the degree of RA patients. But it would get me a chance of heart attack even if my cholesterol was Ok. I am glad now I am lowering my inflammation by avoiding bad foods and eating good foods. This simple habit lowered my inflammation to allow me to enjoy a good healthier life.

To sum up:

New studies for the cause of heart attacks firmly established one thing. It is due to chronic inflammation. From plaque build-up, plaque rupture resulting in clotting at the spot of rupture, it is all due to inflammation. Big clots blocking heart vessels cause heart attacks and strokes.

Cholesterol is used to build the plaque, whether the cholesterol level is high or normal or low. It does not matter. It has been officially declared, "Lowering the cholesterol level does not lower cardiovascular diseases". But lowering inflammation does.

Low-fat diet caused the epidemic of obesity. It is abandoned officially by the government and health organizations. Avoiding saturated fat is still important.

How to lower the inflammation? Please read Chapter 1, and Chapter 42. And Chapter 39 will list most bad foods and good foods.

Chapter Eleven - How my Decades-long Toothache is finally completely gone for now

Dental infections slightly increase the chance of heart attacks (in studies – by 20%)

If you learned what I did, yes, your toothache may be gone too. But you will have a slightly higher chance of a heart attack. From the last chapter, you know chronic inflammation increases the chance of heart attack. Studies in dental sciences have shown that loose teeth with non-healing abscess are foci of infection and source of chronic inflammation. So the proper thing to do is to have the dentist extract the loose teeth, getting rid of the source of infection, if root canal does not help. No matter how small that infection is, some of the researchers insist, even when the loose teeth have no pain, it still increases the chance of heart attack by around 20%.

Frequently brushing teeth lowers the chances of heart attacks? (in studies – by 20% again)

But recent studies also showed brushing teeth three times a day decreased the rate of heart attack by 20% too. Because brushing teeth killed bacteria in the teeth. Otherwise they could get in the blood stream and caused inflammation which in the long run will increase the chance of heart attack, stroke, asthma, arthritis and other chronic diseases that I got rid off as described in this book. So maybe I could keep my loose teeth but make sure I bush teeth at least three times a day. This could cancel the chance of increasing inflammation by loose teeth, because now, the loose teeth don't contain enough bacteria to increase internal inflammation.

How can bacteria in the teeth get into our blood? I learned that as a medical student in NY in the 1970's, a few rigorous walking steps would seed bacteria into our blood streams. (Just imagine scientists doing studies like that. The enrollees were jumping all over the places and then had to have their blood draws to study bacteria in the blood, quite a solemn but active athletic scene. No wonder some people like doing researches.

My toothaches started at grade school

Now back to my toothache story. It began when I was in grade school. One of my left lower molars had an abscess. It hurt so much I could not go to school. I smeared salt around the tooth, slept with it. By the time I woke up. The toothache was gone. That was more than70 years ago, it hurt that much I still remember. (Lots of loud crying too).

I was born and grew up in a poor family, we never had the money for dentistry. I first had my dental visit when I was 21 years old. I started working as a student radiation therapy technologist in Hong Kong. The dental clinic was part of the hospital system. I had two rotten teeth extracted there. That left me with four more loose teeth. They had been giving me toothache pain now and then. But hay, they also gave me the chance of learning how to get rid of toothaches on my own. That was a great chance of serious research, serious learning and serious experimentation. Soon you would find that out.

Aching toothaches finally silenced. Success in experimentation

Finally, I got the pain all controlled ten months ago. Before that, even though with good dental hygiene, the pain has been almost negligible for decades. But the teeth reminded me now and then that they were not normal. Sensitivity or even mild gnawing pain could happen. But now, there is no sensation with hot or cold drinks. No pain on chewing foods, and no pain when not chewing. But now I only have two loose teeth to take care of, one already had a root canal. It was a long fight to keep those teeth for chewing.

The last few paragraphs will detail the various scientifically proven methods to help me turn two rotten teeth that I could extract with my fingers into two firmly planted teeth minus a fistula tract as described in the next chapter.

Milestones in this long experimentation

There were three milestones in the toothache fight that turned the tide to my favorite. The first one was the use of salt. Salt water rinse can mercilessly kill most bacteria in my mouth. I use the rinse once a day in the evening after brushing teeth. Talking about cost-effectiveness, salt is effective and real cheap. The second milestone was when I started brushing teeth after each and every food intake and avoiding sugary food. The third milestone was flossing with toothpaste, or other means to bring toothpaste to between the teeth while simple brushing could not bring toothpaste in those hard-to-reach places so the powerful antibiotics in the toothpaste can work.

Salt kills all kinds of bacteria by osmosis, robbing all the water the bugs have. No living things can live without water

How does salt work? It simply draws all water out from the bacteria by a natural process called osmosis. Without water, the bacteria die their natural deaths. They die by dehydration as the studies showed. We humans can die in seven days too if depleted of water. The researchers reported seeing dead, dehydrated bacterial bodies all over the place. What a fun picture.

Effective as salt was, I still broke out in mild but annoying toothache occasionally, probably because salt follow the path of water. But water cannot penetrate oil. Bacteria hide in films of oil at the gum-line, in the dental pockets. Though, most of the time it worked when I smeared the salt in the loose tooth with pain. Soon, the pain would be gone. But smearing toothpaste with a tooth-pick to the tooth that is aching, the dental pain can be gone faster. The toothpaste is designed to be a powerful mouth bacteria killer.

Tea tree oil and *clove oil* are helpful in controlling toothaches

Tea Tree oil and *clove* oils are so called essential oils (The essence of oils – very concentrated. One little bottle probably takes 60 to 100 pounds of the herbs to make). They are both broad-spectrum antibiotics. They are also strongly antifungal. Clove oil is strongly antiviral, tested effective against skin lesions by HSV-1 (Herpes virus).

If after using salt, the toothache was still there, I used *Tea Tree* oil or *Clove* Oil, applied with a Q-tip around the gum line of the hurting tooth. Don't underestimate the volume of oil in the Q-tip when fully soaked. It was close to 1-cc. I measured it.

Tea Tree oil has strong effect on the central nervous system, be aware

Why did I measure the volume of *Tea Tree* oil in a Q-tip? Was it for the spirit of experimentation? No, because one time 1-cc made me suddenly feeling dizzy for an hour after using *Tea Tree* oil. The dizziness lasted a full hour, though the tooth pain was gone in a few minutes. (No, this experimentation was not that scary compared to some others). I under-estimated the volume of the *Tea Tree* oil in the Q-tips. I did not rinse it off in 10 minutes as I should, estimating it to be just a minute amount. But it was 1-cc as measured later. The 1-cc *Tea Tree* oil was enough to get me dizzy. A few cc (ml) taken by mouth would have put an adult into a deep coma for a few hours, not to say children. A few cc taken internally could be fatal to children. That's how potent the essential oils are.

Another supplement came in handy to fight toothache and periodonitis (inflammation of the gum)

Once I had the toothache, *Tea Tree* oil or *Clove* oil didn't help much, I cut a capsule of the supplement Co-Q 10 and spread the jelly on my gums. Soon, the toothache was gone. I wonder what had happened. Because our body makes Co-Q 10 and it is an enzyme that helped in our body's energy production. Now it made the toothache go away. What explanation I could come up with is a speculation that since the gum tissues are so unhealthy, blood does not readily circulate Co-Q 10 there, and the gum tissues did not have energy for repair. Now Co-Q 10 is rubbed onto the gum, it is fat-soluble, it readily diffuse into gum cells and provide energy for repair.

A dental examination happened days after, and the dentist found the gum tissues were tight around the teeth. The tightness was not present before, I got that feeling of new gum tightness when brushing teeth. I felt the gum-pockets became more firm. So now whenever I feel the gum tissue loose, I would smear the Co-Q 10 jelly from the capsule (as a supplement) onto the gum cells to give them energy to repair.

A similar process happened to the mucous membrane cells in the gut. Leaky gut can repair itself when energy is provided to them in the form of butyrate. Butyrates are short-chain fatty acids generated by gut bacteria eating fibers we cannot digest. That's the main reason we should eat a lot of foods with lots of fibers like green-leaf vegetables which fill half a plate in my meals.

A tiny piece of food will grow million of bacteria

The second mile-stone of learning came during a medical school lecture. I learned that even after tooth brushing and flossing, there could be hundreds of bacteria left, if there is a piece of food as little as a grain of rice left in the mouth. This "food supply" would provide energy for the bacteria to divide every 20 minutes. In a short time, there would be millions and millions of bacteria that are specialists in gum-attack. So since then, I brush teeth meticulously after foods. I usually silently gargle with water for a few minutes to balance the pH of the teeth before brushing. So I won't erode the enamel of the teeth which is soft after food because of the acidity of some foods. I guessed the meticulous brushing greatly slowed down the teeth deterioration with aging. But I rarely would still have mild toothache nevertheless.

Surround your enemies with killing toothpaste on all sides and "fire!"

The third milestone came when my dentist, Dr Enea Bifsha, a smart dentist with a heart in Orlando, Florida, told me to floss with toothpaste when I said I did everything yet still have rare toothaches. That simple act of flossing with toothpaste brought the killing paste to between the teeth. Without doing that, there would not be significant paste between the teeth. I gave it a trial. And gratefully found out it really worked. My toothache has been essentially all gone since then. And if I, on rare occasions, forget to put toothpaste between teeth, a gnawing toothache would come up to bother me. But then if I dip some toothpaste with a tooth-pick and smear it onto where the gum/tooth hurts, the pain would be gone right away. This is like a miracle but not a surprise, because toothpaste is designed to kill oral bacterium.

While I failed to control the annoying mild pain in five long decades, yet this simple act of flossing with toothpaste, or simply stick some toothpaste to where it hurts gently, the pain would vanish in seconds. What was the reason? It seems that the reason is mechanical. The flossing with toothpaste just added strong antibiotics of the toothpaste to between the teeth, which is hard to reach with the brush. When the toothpaste gets in between the teeth, it is like surrounding your enemy (the bacteria) 360 degrees with lethal weapons firing. They will die readily, though somewhat reluctantly.

Toothpaste-bubbles don't do the job, it needs real paste

Perhaps I should add another important learning along with the learning of toothpaste-flossing. This one was not learned from a great dentist. I learned it from the writing on a tube of toothpaste. It tells me that I should apply real toothpaste to every tooth, instead of just spreading the bubbles created by water. So toothpaste bubbles don't work, beware! So I put a little bit of the paste onto the brush, four to six times, to each tooth at the gum lines of only a few teeth till all the teeth are covered. So enough toothpaste at the right spots does matter a lot.

Just like that, my 50 years of occasional toothache or tooth sensitivity was gone. It's gone for about a year now.

Dentist certified that my two loose teeth no long needed extraction

Half a year ago, two of my teeth were so loose that I could almost pulled them out easily with my fingers only. So teeth extraction was about to be scheduled, but I was going North to New York for the summer. So we put off the extraction, and I decided to work on the teeth to see if I could strengthen them back firmly on solid grounds of the strengthened bones and gums.

To heal these two teeth, I planned four things and really seriously carried them out in this teeth-saving experiment.

First, I had to restore my immune system so it can help heal the infection at the root of the pre-molar. My immune system was indeed getting stronger while I continued my active healthy life style, started eating the Paleo-like/ Mediterranean diet. The increased immune attack on the bacteria would be from the inside of the teeth out.

Secondly, I would make sure the sick teeth were bathed in toothpaste each time I brushed my teeth. The toothpaste would attack the bacteria from outside in. It became possible then for the toothpaste to reach from the outside to the inside of the tooth at the root since the drainage was through the pockets surrounding the tooth. Enough toothpaste used is very important. In the past, I underused the toothpaste, thinking the bubbles created by the meager amount of paste were enough like soup bubbles. Now, to have enough paste, I reapply a bit of paste every few teeth.

Thirdly, I had to supply my teeth with vitamin C, calcium, vitamin D and phosphorus to build the enamel. So I started taking calcium 600 mg a day, Vitamin D 200 IU a day, and increase my daily meat, nuts intake for phosphorus. Vitamin C was 1000 mg I took every other day. That dose was plenty. The vitamin C is against the damaging effect of the fluoride added in water. The vitamin D, calcium, and phosphorus are used to build up the bone of the teeth. So the enamel could grow and hold on to the pins from the top half of the tooth more tightly. That tooth was broken twenty years ago. Another dentist with a heart in California spent a whole hour and fixed the top half back to the root-half with two pins. Talking devotion to patients, dentists and doctors sometimes are alike and usually they are honored with 5-stars.

Fourthly, I flossed with toothpaste (See Chapter Eleven for details), so I could surround the sick teeth on all sides, not just the outside, but also between the teeth. So after brushing teeth, I flossed before gargle with water so I can floss with toothpaste. In this way, the powerful bacterial-killing power of the toothpaste would kill the bacteria from outside in, surrounding the teeth for a few minutes to do the killing of bacteria.

I diligently carried out the tasks I needed to do to save these teeth. I restored my healthy immune system (see Chapter One), brushed teeth after food each time with plenty of toothpaste to kill bacteria in hard to reach places, taking vitamin C, calcium, vitamin D, and phosphorus (in meat and nuts etc) to build the hardness for the enamel of the tooth, flossing with toothpaste before the gargling with water, three times a day.

In three months in the summer of 2019. My premolar became brand new. Infection became minimal. The molar became firm, and the top half tightly pinned onto the base. The pre-molar had been saved, the fistula no longer appeared. Mission Impossible accomplished. The habits that helped restored the health of this teeth became a daily routine. All I have to do is to continue for the rest of my life. Yes it is troublesome, but I have to do it. I was glad there was another set of smart life-styling habits gained!

Half a year later, after I brushed teeth after each meal carefully following what I described above, the two previously loose teeth became more firm and pain-free and became insensitive on chewing. I finally went back to Dr Bifsha for dental check-up and cleaning. After a careful professional examination, he declared my teeth no longer needed extraction. Was I glad to hear the result of the examination!

Now I could keep those teeth essential for chewing. Just imagine all the good foods in the world waiting for me to chew on, you could feel my gratitude and joy. Yes, I am counting the good foods in my mind now.

Brief discussions of the herbs used in this chapter

1. *Tea Tree* oil is from a small tree different from the shrubs that produce tea for drinking. It is a very popular essential oil. One little bottle of it is "distilled" from probably 60 pounds of the *Tea Tree* leaves and branch-tips. It is not that caustic, I applied it undiluted, though most gurus advised diluting it with olive oil or other oils before use. It is strictly for external use only. A few cc taken internally will put an adult into coma for a few hours. It has been extensively used in acne for its antibacterial effects. It may irritate the skin in sensitive people.

2. *Clove* oil is multifunctional too. But it is the most popular oil for toothache. *Clove* oil is a constituent in "Tiger Balm" that the Chinese and Asian people used for fever, cold and other ailments. For more side effects and other uses please see PDR for Herbal Medicine in every public library.

    Clove oil topically smeared on skin or gum can get nasty side effects of gum-bleeding in sensitive people.

    A case report in PDR for Herbal Medicine described a college student smoked *clove* cigarette and died of bleeding in the lungs and respiratory failure.

    Otherwise *clove* oil is relatively safe if used properly.

Last, but not the least

Not enough sleep can weaken our immunity outright. Just a week ago, I stayed up late writing this book, and the toothache returned. My weakened immunity due to the lack of sleep allowed the bad bugs to flourish, and attacked my gums causing pain. For the next 4 days, I had to get more rest and eventually the toothache quiet down.

This reminded me why young doctors and nurses unfortunately died in this current Respiratory virus pandemic. They were in the frontline trying to save patients from the Respiratory virus pandemic, and they overworked, not getting enough sleep, and weakened their immunity and they died like elderly people whose immunity is weak for various lifestyle problems.

To sum up:

Extraction of very loose teeth refractory to treatments would lower the chance of heart attacks as new studies showed. And this is the proper dental treatment. But brushing teeth three times a day decrease the risk of heart attack by the same percentage. So I am keeping my two loose teeth, and brush my teeth after eating any food when I am at home. If out in restaurants, I gargle with water many times, and used tooth picks in the men's room to clean teeth if there is privacy. Please let your teeth be extracted if necessary. I have to keep the two slightly loose teeth because without them, I cannot chew.

So extraction was not a good option. Though I had to work hard to try to keep my teeth clean and hoped to get rid of the toothaches and hoped the loose teeth would last forever. I brushed teeth three times a day with copious amount of toothpaste since they are designed to kill bacteria in the mouth. I flossed while the teeth were all immersed in toothpaste before I brush so maximum amount of toothpaste is still there.

When there was toothache, salt smeared to the tooth helped. Rinsing with salt-water would help to get rid of the pain. If that failed, I use *Tea Tree* oil or *Clove* oil on a Q-tube and apply it topically. They are toxic. Both have to be rinsed off in 10 minutes. Rinsing off is very necessary because those oils are very toxic if they got absorbed into the body. A few milliliter (ml) of Tea Tree oil can be fatal for children if swallowed. This same amount swallowed can put an adult into coma too.

So "flossing with toothpaste" was the final solution. I am free of toothache after I added that. It worked after I apply toothpaste onto my teeth, then I flossed. But I made sure that what I put on my teeth was the paste, not the bubbles created by water.

Chapter Twelve - Loose Teeth and Fistula Tract fixed

Success in eliminating a fistula (tunnel) with a supplement

In March, 2019, one of my teeth was in big trouble. It was extremely loose. It could be moved back and forth with a light touch. It could be slided up and down from the base. This tooth was the pre-molar on the upper jaw on my right side. It is one of the teeth that grinds the food for me. It is the only grinding mortar I have. 20 years ago in California, its top half broke off from the base. Two pins put it back to the base by a dentist with a big heart, patience and delicate skills (It took a long time to fix that tooth).

At this time in March, 2020, it could slide up and down of the pin holes easily. I decided to keep it and try to heal it. But by healing the fistula, blocking the exit of the edema fluid, I put the poor tooth in this precarious condition myself. The fluid drained through the pre-molar base instead, loosening it. I got to fix it because it is the main tooth in my only chewing mortar. And it took the California 5-stars dentist more than an hour to fix. I got to treasure it.

Two months ago in January, 2019, I got rid of a fistula (tunnel) connecting the deep root of this infected pre-molar tooth through the gum of the next tooth and empty the edema fluid out into the mouth. The edema fluid was due to the infection at the root of the pre-molar. It only accumulated rarely to drain. But the infection was persistent for the past ten years, despite a root canal cleaning and sealing, and multiple bouts of antibiotics.

I hated the fistula on my gum. I could feel it with my finger running from the pre-molar to the gum of the next tooth. It popped out now and then rarely. It was a big source of inflammation and pain, especially right before it was ready to burst. So I decided to get rid of the fistula. I learned that CO-Q10, a natural co-enzyme in our body, also available as a supplement, could strengthen the gum, tighten the dental pockets and it just might heal the fistula.

Co-Q 10 is an integral part of the inner membrane of mitochondria in our cells. Mitochondrias are the energy factories in our cells. When there is no energy supply, the gum cells cannot mend itself. It is known that a deficiency of Co-Q 10 can cause periodontitis, the inflammation in the gum around the root of the teeth.

So I bought the CO-Q 10 supplement online. It came in capsules. Cutting the top of the capsule, I squeezed the pinkish gel onto my clean index finger, spread it along the inside and outside of the gum. I did it twice a day for 3 days. Sure enough, the fistula was gone. The scientific explanation was proposed in the last chapter. I would not repeat here.

I was happy, not knowing I was going to get a big surprise from sealing the fistula by tightening the gum tissue. Because then the edema fluid had nowhere to drain when in rare occasions the inflammation flares up. Then it could only drain through its own gum pockets surrounding the root of the pre-molar tooth.

Success came at a price

What happened was then the edema fluid from the pre-molar infection drained through the pockets of its own tooth. These "pockets" surrounded the tooth. The draining fluid loosened up the pre-molar, almost pushed the top piece of the tooth off. The dental hygienist and the dentist in Florida were adversely impressed. They pronounced the two teeth officially dead and advised extractions. I stealthily escaped to New York to have more time to heal the teeth. To be honest, we usually spend time in New York with the grandchildren in the summer months, so I just packed up and drove to New York, with the pre-molars in their sockets loosely, bouncing up and down in their sockets while I was driving along I-95N.

Because I have to keep these teeth in, so I could chew hard foods like nuts. Nuts like walnuts, macadamia nuts and pecan nuts, have a lot of protein, fibers, resistant starch, and good fats, the omega-3. Omega-3 is an anti-inflammatory good fatty acid. Most other nuts have a lot more omega-6 than omega-3. Omega-6 is inflammatory. But all the nuts still have plenty of proteins and fibers, vitamins and minerals—enough to grow a tree. Even though most nuts besides those mentioned above, have more omega-6, and thus could be inflammatory if eaten. But it may be Ok to be consumed if taken together with plenty of non-starchy vegetables and good proteins, which are anti-inflammatory. I eat a few walnuts when I am hungry between meals, just a few walnuts and no more. It is filling and is a very good food with pretty dense calories. This is a recommendable way of losing weight, eating a few nuts when hungry between meals, but no more than a few.

Complicated scheme to save the teeth for the keeping as long as I can

To heal these two teeth, I planned four things and really did it. Let me repeat the methods now in this chapter that I said in the last chapter for people who skipped the good information.

First, I had to restore my immune system so it can help heal the infection at the root of the pre-molar. My immune system was indeed getting stronger while I continued my active healthy life style, started eating the Paleo-like/ Mediterranean diet. The stronger immune attack on the bacteria would be from the inside of the pre-molar teeth out.

Secondly, I would make sure the sick teeth were bathed in toothpaste each time I brushed my teeth. The toothpaste with its custom made antibiotics for the mouth bacteria, would attack the bacteria from outside in. It became possible then to reach the root of the tooth from outside since the drainage was through the pockets surrounding the tooth. Enough toothpaste used is very important. In the past, I underused the toothpaste, thinking the bubbles created by the meager amount of paste and water was the real paste. To have enough paste, I reapply the paste every few teeth.

Thirdly, I had to supply my teeth with vitamin C, calcium, vitamin D and phosphorus to build the enamel, the bone of the tooth. So I started taking calcium 600 mg a day, Vitamin D 200 IU a day, and increase my daily meat and nuts intake to get enough phosphorus. Vitamin C was 1000 mg I took every other day. That dose was plenty. The vitamin C is against the discoloring effect of the fluoride added in water. The vitamin D, calcium, and phosphorus are used to build up the bone of the teeth. So the enamel could grow and hold on to the pins from the top half of the tooth more tightly.

Fourthly, I flossed with toothpaste, so I could surround the sick teeth on all sides, not just the outside and inside, but also between the teeth. So after brushing teeth, I flossed before gargle with water that clears the paste away. In this way, the powerful bacterial-killing power of the toothpaste would kill the bacteria from outside in, surrounding the teeth for a few minutes to do the killing of bacteria that the toothpaste was designed to do.

I diligently carried out the tasks I needed to do to save these teeth. I restored my healthy immune system as said in Chapter One, brushed teeth after food each time with plenty of toothpaste, taking vitamin C, calcium, vitamin D, and phosphorus (in meat and nuts etc), flossing with toothpaste before gargling with water, three times a day.

In three months in the summer of 2019. My premolars became brand new. Infection became minimal. The molar became firm, and the top half tightly pinned onto the base. The pre-molar had been saved, the fistula no longer appeared. Mission Impossible accomplished.

Routine immune control on the bacteria in the pre-molar included adequate sleeping time

Not enough sleep can weaken our immunity outright. Studies have shown if the sleeping time is less than five hours, the most numerous white blood cells, the neutrophils that fight bacteria, lost a lot of its function in sleep-deprivation. The immune system right there was much weaker. Just a week ago, I stayed up late writing this book, and the toothache returned. I could feel the shortened fistula coming back. It did not reach the gum of the next tooth like it was, before I "fixed' it. Because I used CO-Q 10 to build up the "muscles" of the next tooth that the fistula used to drain out to the oral cavity. So there was no fistula anymore but an edematous base of the pre-molar. My weakened immunity due to the lack of sleep allowed the bad bugs to flourish, and attacked my gums causing pain, causing edema fluid to accumulate at the base of the premolar. For the next 4 days, I had to get more rest and eventually the toothache quiet down. The edema disappeared.

One needs six to eight hours of sleeping time to keep the immune system happy.

To sum up -

I need to keep my right upper pre-molar. It is an essential tooth I cannot do without. It was loosened by the drainage fluid from the infection inside. I fixed a fistula connected to the root of the molar to an opening in the gum tissue of the next tooth. I tightened the gum tissue and closed the fistula off. Months before, CO-Q 10 was used, sealing its drainage canal. The re-routed

drainage, after the fistula was sealed, drained through the pre-molar itself weakened the pre-molar tooth, even though it only happened very rarely.

To save the tooth, I attacked the bacteria at the root of the tooth with an enhanced immune system (see Chapter One). It attacked the bacteria from inside out. I use more toothpaste than before, and smeared the paste between teeth with flossing when brushing teeth, or I used a tooth pick, dipped some toothpaste and smeared it where it hurt, to kill the bacteria from outside right away with the pain gone almost instantly. So the application of toothpaste directly on the spot that hurts really kills the offending bacteria out right.

I took vitamin D, calcium and more phosphorus from food to build up the enamel. In three months, a new tooth was "re-furbished", it was firmer with solid enamel holding tightly to the pins of the upper half of the broken tooth. Even though now it remained a slightly infected one, that perhaps I could chew with for a long time. And my renewed immune system should be able to decrease the size of the molar infection and there was no more edema fluid.

At the same time, I have to have enough sleeping time to keep my immune system strong so the pre-molar infection can be contained effectively. Removing it will terminate the infection focus, but a replacement false-tooth would not be strong enough to chew hard foods like nuts, which is a key food for me to keep slim and strong. (Eating nuts often will give me the good fats and proteins I need badly to boost my metabolic rate and keep from getting obese, if I limit myself to ONLY a handful of it).

Chapter Thirteen - How I lowered my Risk of Colon Cancers

All colon cancer started as polyps, so to prevent colon cancers is to prevent polyps

Most cancers are not hereditary (only 3 to 5% are). Then how did I know I had a higher risk of colon cancer? For one thing, I had Irritable Bowel Syndrome though not a bad one. Irritable Bowel Syndrome (IBS) gives eight folds the chance of colon cancers. So it was not to my surprise in finding that years ago, there was a small polyp by colonoscopy in my colon, making the risk of colon cancer higher. It is believe all colon cancers started as polyps in the background of inflammation. Colonoscopy showed my colon was inflamed. Though only the big polyps or special type of polyps do have the chance to become cancers.

Polyps grow only slowly, so colonoscopy every three to five years will catch them in time and remove them through colonoscopies. (Some situations may call for more frequent colonoscopies). It was painless to me, because I was under anesthesia. That is, I was totally numbed up.

My higher risk of colon cancer foretold by a psychic (Who is not a gut specialist MD)

But what made the chance of colon cancer most likely? It was made very likely by the words of a psychic, a friend's advice/prediction. He could communicate with souls or people from another physical dimension. More than ten years ago, he told me in my later life, I would have "trouble" with my bowels and I should make a vegetable smoothie with a blender to drink every morning. I tried to drink vegetable smoothie every morning, but developed diarrheas. So I turned to eating a lot of cooked vegetables daily. The psychic's words was valuable, soon colonoscopy showed I had a polyp.

Are there people from another dimension the psychic can communicate with, really? Yes. Am I crazy? No, I learned this in "physics" in one of the city-colleges, of the City University of New York. It was close to Memorial Sloan-Kettering Cancer Center where I worked as a radiation therapy technologist in the daytime, attending college in the evening. In fact, this "4th dimension" was one of Albert Einstein's theories. So another dimension does exist. No doubt about it, since Einstein said it.

But this 4th dimension can be spiritual rather than physical. One day, maybe each of us shall find out just what that particular dimension is when we finally would float through a tunnel with bright light at the end of that tunnel (i.e. when we die). Out of the tunnel into another dimension is a very attractive idea to a man with boundless curiosity like me, though I am not in any hurry to find out. Why? because there is a good book for me to write.

With the discovery of a polyp in my colonoscopy, I know I do have a higher chance of getting colon cancers. But I know chances are I won't get one, because I know how to prevent cancers. Why? How do I know? Because I wrote the books on cancer preventions! (Please pardon my humor. But I do sincerely believe the information in my other 3 books would help prevent cancers or prevent its recurrence. All the three books are being sold at cost, on-line).

Lots of fibers in foods lower the chance of colon cancers

From my prior medical school learning in NY, I already knew lots of fibers are found in the vegetables. And that "lots of fibers in food" lowers the chance of colon cancer. In the 1960's, it was found out that people in Africa had a lot lower incidence of colon cancers because their foods had a lot of fibers. (That was a thing of the past, now their foods are fast affected by Western fast-foods and processed foods).Vegetables have eight times the fiber-contents than commercial preparations weight for weight, even the fruits have twice the fiber contents. This was written in books.

With the psychic's dire warning in my mind and the fear of cancer in my heart, I dug deeper in the search of knowledge to fan off the colon cancer by destiny.

Next in line I had to do was to get rid of my Irritable Bowel Syndrome which is associated with eight time higher risk of colon cancer. So foods that send me to the bathroom for diarrhea got eliminated from my diet one by one: Most fresh fruits, milk and cheese, wheat products with gluten like bread, cookies, cakes, biscuits, croissants, muffins, coffees, teas, sugar, and sweeteners. Sugar causes inflammation in the body because high concentration in the blood will generate free radicals. Radicals are charged particles in blood that cause inflammations. So I found *Stevia* (pronounced stee've ah). It is a plant that makes our taste bud to say, "Ah, sugar!" but it is really not sugar. It was declared non-cancer causing officially by studies. I enjoyed it with coconut milk tea. Yes, I should stay away from tea. But green teas don't give me diarrheas. We are just humans, aren't we all? I drank green tea quite often.

Since fresh vegetables also gave me diarrhea. I cooked them well so they would not give me diarrhea. So the perfect plate of food for me is half a plate of cooked vegetable, with the other half being good proteins and good fats like avocados, nuts and seeds, chicken, fish, sea foods, or grass-fed beef. That should keep my inflammation down and not resulting in any diarrhea, no? Not yet. Eating 80% full is the key to avoid inflammation and chronic diseases. In other words, if you eat till you feel 100% full, you are actually 120% full, and those excess calories will be converted to fats in the liver. Fats cells secret all kind of inflammatory chemicals and bring us the internal inflammation.

It takes 20 minutes for the stomach to tell the brain," I'm full, master, please give order to stop eating".

No, if I eat till 100% full, then I would have been over-eating. The extra calorie would turn into fat. Fat cells make all kinds of inflammatory molecules like IL-6 and TNF-alpha (IL-interleukin, TNF-tumor necrosis factor). These chemicals will eventually bring back my Irritable Bowel Syndrome and bring diarrheas and increase the risk of colon cancer in the long run. So I stop eating when just feeling a little full, or before I feel full. The stomach's "full" signal won't reach the brain till 20 minutes later. In 20 minutes, we will be eating excess calories that the body will store as fat, most likely in our bellies.

Loosing weight would lose the fat. Good proteins and good fats on the plates help us lose weight, they speed up metabolism, not starchy carbohydrates like potatoes which slow down metabolism (Tested, all done by breathe-test of CO_2). The excess 20% carbohydrates could get turned into fats in the liver. This is responsible for the 60% of Americans being over-weight. Low fat diet (but high carbohydrate) was the reason two generations of us gained too much weight. Now low fat diet is abandoned by all health authorities and organizations. Good fats and good proteins are the healthy foods that are going to stay. Their staying power comes from thousands of research studies. On the other hand, low fat diet messed us up because it was based on just a few poorly run studies.

The real important intervention that allows me to get rid of my IBS is the simple act of avoiding bad foods and eating good foods and eating 80% full. The explanation is long. It was presented in Chapter 9. In short, good foods heal our leaky gut walls, stop the millions of antigens (foreign particles) from going into our circulation to cause our immune-system to be dysfunctional and cause chronic inflammation in our body. The inflammation also occurs in our gut and at the gut walls. No inflammation, no damaged gut walls, and diarrhea stops. Life is just so mechanical. I realized that life, being so complicated, mysterious, romantic, glorious, but after all, is very mechanical, especially from molecular biology points of view.

So I am looking forward to a life with lower risk of colon cancers. Thanks to the psychic friend for reminding me of my lousy destiny which, after all, seems alterable.

Some supplements I am taking may lower my risk of colon cancers also on the long run, as prevention.

There must be hundreds of supplements that were tested to lower cancers in the laboratory or in studies analyzing population of peoples or in animal studies. But when people take those supplements, they still get cancer. In fact, if one is not deficient, regular dose of vitamins or supplements could bring a higher risk of cancers. Also is taking superfluous supplements. Those were the very reliable findings from "golden studies". So take them only if you need them.

Generally speaking, eating healthy foods and living healthy life-styles will greatly lower the risk of cancers. Exercise being the strongest of the "supplement-life style" that really minimize the chance of cancer. In "golden studies", exercise can lower the risk of cancers by 40%. But I think equally important, if not more important, is tending to gut health to restore the potency of the immune system to prevent cancer. This trumps it all, without any doubt. But some supplements I am taking for other reasons, had been studied and found to prevent cancer. But of course I do not depend much on them at all to prevent cancer.

Ginkgo biloba I am taking for tinnitus (ringing in the ear) and fortuitously found to help control my ED was found in studies to lower the risk of ovarian cancers. The lutein I am taking for my vision sharpness was studied and found to prevent quite a few kind of cancers like lung, breast, prostate, endometrial cancer, and ovarian cancers. Lutein can modulate immune response. Given to cats, lutein was found to increase the helper- cells which are cancer killing cells, called CD4 lymphocytes (a kind of white blood cells). Even the calcium I am taking for bone health and dental-health, was found to possibly able to prevent colon cancer. They might help, but only very little help compared to the force of restoring the potency of the immune system (Chapter 50 may have more details).

Last of all, probiotics in fermented milk was found to prevent some bladder cancers from coming back in a human study. The patients who did not drink fermented milk had more bladder cancers again in that control study. This study was done in the real world in humans in intervention style who had bladder cancers treated before. So tending to the gut health with probiotics would really seem to strengthen the immune system against cancers, at least bladder cancers.

To sum up -

I was fortunate to have a psychic friend to tell me to avoid colon cancer when I get old. I did reshape a few life-habits to try to lower my risk of colon cancer. To be real, colonoscopy at the appropriate time will detect polyps which if they are big or bad types, can turn into colon cancers. So colonoscopies have been found to save lives from colon cancer in studies. There are additional ways to lower colon cancers.

The first was from medical school learning. To eat a lot of non-starchy vegetables to create "bulk" in the colon, that is: lots of fibers. Because fibers can heal a leaky gut wall, because fibers that we cannot digest, the gut bacteria turned them into short chain fatty acids that will serve as energy source for our gut cells to repair themselves so they will heal the leaky guts, that eventually stops my IBS. (The good gut bacteria turned fibers into butyrate to mend the gut wall). IBS is associated with 8 times the risk of colon cancer.

Secondly is to avoid any food that causes me to have a stomach-upset. They could hurt my gastrointestinal system,

increasing the risk of cancer.

Thirdly is to control my weight, to lower the inflammation in my body. Losing weight by losing fat cells will lower the internal inflammations and thus lowers the risk of colon cancer.

Fourthly is to avoid bad foods and eat good foods, (Chapter 39). My immune system will be strong and probably should prevent colon cancer or other cancers. This is one of the wonders of healing the gut to strengthen the immune system or restoring the potency of the immune system against cancers. Taking probiotics (beneficial bacteria commercially available) perhaps may turn out to be a potent supplementation to keep the immune system perfect, and keep my health in top shape. But it needs more studies.

But the most important weapons to fight to prevent colon cancer are the idea to boost my body-power. Conventional cancer treatments do not include the body-power. But scientific studies, hundreds of them, did show boosting the body-power can dwarf cancer. So I added smart lifestyles to boost body-power to help fight cancers. It worked. From my experience of treating thousands of cancer patients before I retired, patients with early stage cancers I treated never recurred, as I remember. The late stage cancer patients stretched their time from one year to 3 or 5 years. These life saving life-style tips are *exercise, eat till 80% full, relieve stress, no sugar, don't gain weight, eat lots of non-starchy vegetables and avoid saturated fats*.

I definitely will include these weapons to prevent the colon cancer that is destined to happen in me.

Chapter Fourteen –

How one old Friend lived 4 Years instead of 1 Year with an end-stage Lung Cancer metastatic to the Bones and Liver at Diagnosis

- A sad case of lung cancer -

My heart is still aching from a friend's death in the spring of 2019. She was an accountant living in Los Angelis (L.A.). She was diagnosed of lung cancer in 2015. At the time of diagnosis, it already involved the bones, the liver, and probably the brain. Her oncologist in LA kindly gave an estimation of survival to be 10 months. I am an oncologist too. I think the estimate was on the kind side. This lady accountant was my high school classmate in Hong Kong. In fact, in grade 1, she sat with my wife, sharing the same desk. So our friendship went back for about than 70 years.

I would guess the survival after diagnosis in a case like hers would be only 6 to 8 months. Another high school classmate's wife was diagnosed of lung cancer at a late stage like this classmate of ours, just was able to live for about 6 months. That's what it is. Lung cancer at late stage is really bad. On the other hand, a certain percent of patients with early stages of lung cancers can be cured.

With my oncology (cancer treatment) experience, I thought I should be able to help. Did I?

Right after diagnosis, she got in touch with me by phone, from LA to New York. She was desperate. She read all my books cover to cover and over again. The first three books I wrote were all about cancer control. It was from my experience of treating thousands of cancer patients before I retired. They are being sold at cost online.

Why did my cancer patients do better than the average patients?

From the last chapter, I mentioned boosting body-power to add to the power of the conventional anti-cancer therapy. My cancer patients did a lot better than the average. Patients with early stage cancers I treated never recurred, as I remember. The late stage cancer patients stretched their time from one year to 3 or 5 years. Almost all the cancer patients I treated benefited from the smart life-styling I taught them. These are *exercise, eat till 80% full, relieve stress, no sugar, don't gain weight, eat plenty of non-starchy vegetables, and avoid saturated fats.* Let me explain a little more:

.Exercise: Long known to enhance the immune system. It boosts immune system by various means. It was all from studies. The underlying sciences will be elaborated in Part Two of this book in Chapter 45 or in my other three books being sold at cost online.

.Eat till 80% full: It takes 20 minutes for an already full stomach to tell the brain to stop eating. If you eat till full. You eat too much. Gaining weight in studies was shown to weaken the immune system. On the other hand, active weight-loss strengthens the immune system.

.Relieve stress: Stress increase inflammation in our body. Blood test will show their presence. Inflammation from stress weakens the immune system. Key immune cells fighting bacteria and cancer went down by 70% in the seemingly harmless stress brought by sleep deprivation. Adequate sound sleep is a strong stress-buster and immune-booster.

.No sugar - Americans eat the most calories from sugar, from a Tuft University study. The sugar is in the form of high fructose corn syrup (HFCS) which is the sugar in all processed foods. Why is it bad? HFCS is sugar. Sugar is inflammatory. It is also the only one fuel for cancer cells. Excess sugar turned into fat. Fat cells secretes inflammatory chemicals to increase the internal inflammations

.Keep the same weight (i.e. don't gain weight). Weight gain means gaining fats. Fat cells make inflammatory chemicals. Inflammation weakens the immune system.

.Eat plenty of vegetables – Fibers in vegetables will heal out guts and improve the immune system against cancer recurrence.

.Avoid saturated fats – It increase inflammation and weakens the immunity.

Do the above smart habits really boost the immune system enough to fight cancer?

Indeed, thanks to the same smart habits, one of my patients did have her carcinoid (meaning a little cancer) cured from her lung. For months, she worked hard at those lifestyle habits just mentioned and lost 3 pounds by six months follow up. She restored her immune potency with the smart life-styling. The smart habits enabled her to shred 3 pounds. Her immune system improved enough to get rid of the "little cancer". In the six months follow up, the carcinoid was gone from her lung seen from computed tomography (CT).

A good immune system is enough to prevent cancer or even get rid of a "little cancer". How about a real bad cancer? Good question. The answer is affirmative. A good immune system can even cure a deadly very aggressive cancer.

A restored strong immune system was able to get rid of an aggressive cancer

When cancer happens, it is generally believed that there probably are some defects in the immune system. Restoring the potency of the immune system may get rid of a real fatal cancer as in Molly's case discussed in Chapter One. (Please see Chapter One for this real interesting case). But I will summarize it here. Molly was a 3-years old little girl with leaky guts due to celiac disease. Her immune system was dysfunctional due to the leaky guts. Kaposi's sarcoma, a deadly cancer, was found in her right eye.

But the normal functioning immune system is capable of immune-surveillance against cancer cells. Once the surveillance cells found those cancer cells, they will label the cells and signal the soldiers (cells) to kill the cancer cells. Molly was eventually cured of a fatal Kaposi's sarcoma in her right eye. The cancer started when she had leaky guts leading to dysfunctional immune system allowing cancer to grow. She healed her leaky guts due to celiac disease. The good gut-wall now prevented foreign particles to get in her circulation to make the immune system dysfunctional. After the gut wall was repaired by avoiding gluten foods. Her immune system resumed its potent function, and killed the Kaposi's sarcoma. I wish in this way, all cancers can be cured. I kind of doubt it but there is no study to say this cannot be done.

Unfortunately, advanced lung cancer not controlled by the old immune system in this case

This high school classmate was virtually sentenced to death by cancer in 10 months. The world cannot be crueler than that. How unlucky she was. I have not learned the gut-healing diet related to the potency of the immune system yet. I learned it a year too late for this classmate. How I wish I had learned it just a year earlier.

If she learned the diet-immune system relationship, she would certainly try eating good foods, avoiding bad foods. Like Molly curing her sarcoma by her restored immune system, my classmate might have gained 5 to 10 years instead. A restored immune system for her should be able to lengthen her life more. That is highly possible. Then, may be then, her almost 100 years old mom wouldn't be so heart-broken when my high school classmate eventually died in her sleep in the Spring of 2019, 4 years after the diagnosis of her lung cancer. This was cruelly devastating to her elderly mom, like any parent in the world, to have seen their kids die. I think this was the ultimate pain for my classmate and for her mom. My classmate's only wish for herself was to outlive her mom but she couldn't!

Nevertheless, there was great consolation to me. With the smart life-styling knowledge I dug out from research studies and written into previous three books. She studied them hard and formed good cancer surviving habits. This greatly helped her cutting-edge molecular cancer treatment the oncologist in LA was giving her. She lasted almost four good years. Those were very good years. She toured a lot of places in the world with other classmates in the West Coast. Life was almost normal. Those were four good years.

Shared knowledge of cancer fighting habits benefited her friends too

She told me several of her fellow patients from the same support group, having end-stage cancers like her, shared the same smart habits recommended in my books. Together they lived longer like herself. Not all other patients with advanced stage cancers outside of their group. They lasted only a few months. Some would live a few more months if the cancer burden was lighter. But none of the advanced stage cancer patients lived like her group sharing the smart life habits. She was secretly very happy they all lived years longer, she told me in one of our numerous phone conversations. The fact that she lived 3.5 years longer is still a good consolation for me.

How I wished I learned the gut-immune system connection just a year earlier. Our classmate of 70 years might still be alive. This crushed wish always makes me want to cry.

To sum up:

A high school classmate, a friend of my wife since grade 1, had late stage lung cancer. She was given 10 months to live, as estimated by her oncologist in LA. She lived four normal years with the knowledge from my previous three books. This knowledge was a potent weapon in the fight against cancer. It described about seven lifestyle habits to strengthen one's body against cancer. She and several of her fellow patients in the same support group lived years longer with this knowledge, compared to others outside their group.

Conventional cancer treatments do not include the body-power. But scientific studies, hundreds of them, did show boosting the body-power can dwarf cancer. So I added smart lifestyles to boost body-power to help fight cancers. It worked. From my experience of treating thousands of cancer patients before I retired, patients with early stage cancers I treated never recurred, as I remember. The late stage cancer patients stretched their time from one year to 3 or 5 years. Almost all of them were benefited from the smart life-styling I taught them. These life saving life-style tips are *exercise, eat till 80% full, relieve stress, no sugar, don't gain weight, eat lots of non-starchy vegetables and avoid saturated fats.*

But further new knowledge of healing the leaky guts, restoring the potent function of the immune system, getting rid of a deadly cancer like in Molly's case, came too late for my classmate with lung cancer.

Yes this new knowledge I learned was too late for this long time classmate, but hopefully it is not too late for others.

Chapter Fifteen - My Dry-Eyes do not need Eye-Drops anymore

Dry eyes bothered me all my life

Dried eyes were a lot of inconvenience to me. All my life, my eyes got tired after reading for about 30 minutes. My eyes felt dry and tired, even as I squinted my eyes tight, no tears could be squeezed out to my rescue. Thankfully, eye-drops worked, so I used it several times a day. But the problem was, most of the time, I did not have this little bottle of eye-drops in my pockets. That was inconvenient, especially when I was in my office, reading patients' charts in the computer screen. Reading became a struggle on rare occasions. I still remembered the frustration. It is different now. I am glad I can read well for 1 to 2 hours with naturally lubricated eyes now, before I have to rest my eyes. Such nice-reading times have happened recently for about half a year. Now I have no need for eye-drops.

The fact that my pair of eyes is so well naturally lubricated is new in my life. I was using my eyes without realizing I did not need eye-drops for almost half a year before it finally dawned on me. I don't need eye-drops anymore. Now and then I still see those little bottles of eye-drops laying in every corner of the house and how I wished they could be refunded for money.

Dry-eyes disappeared as chronic inflammation goes down

What happened? Why should the dry-eyes go away by themselves? Were there any aliens involved? Finally, readings in the Functional Medicine gurus' books revealed that as the inflammation went down, dry-eyes problem would resolve in no time too. No wonder, it is just one of the chronic diseases that would disappear. I just avoided the inflammatory foods, my dry-eyes have become dry no more. Then I looked back in the past few months what foods I eat, what foods I avoided.

The bad foods I avoided, not even a 100% half the time, yet that was good enough. These are foods that most people are sensitive to, but probably not knowing it themselves. The "side effects" (manifestations) of eating them are chronic diseases. So anybody with chronic diseases should suspect inflammation inside and should give a trial of avoiding bad foods to see if their chronic diseases go away or not.

Foods that cause inflammation

The major inflammatory foods for 80% of the people, is gluten containing foods. Gluten contains 40 proteins found in wheat, rye, barley, and oats contaminated in the factories where wheat products are also manufactured. Though only 5% people are seriously sensitive to gluten, which can damage their guts causing celiac disease with symptoms of fatigue, weight loss, diarrhea or constipation, but 80% of us are sensitive to gluten and got damages to a lesser degree. It is worthwhile to mention that because bad foods results in internal inflammation which brings all kinds of chronic diseases including dry eyes. That is why everybody is avoiding gluten nowadays.

Other foods as inflammatory as gluten include milk, cheese, and lots of sugar. Sugar is in every processed food. To make processed foods tasty, there is one golden rule for the manufacturers. It is to use lots of sugar, salt and butter (fats). So the food can taste delicious and be able to hook us up. You may not believe it. Hooking us up is the primary goal of processed foods manufacturers. Do I mind being hooked up by food? Yes, very much. I just don't want to be hooked up by inflammatory foods and bust my immune system.

Gluten is present in wheat, rye, barley, oats etc and even in some antiseptic hand-sanitizer foams and cosmetics. There is going to be more to say about gluten in Chapter 39, Good Foods and Bad Foods.

Dry eyes disappeared as my allergy went away

There is no mystery here. As my allergy went away after the restoration of my immune system was achieved. I have no need for antihistamine. And the immune system is calmed but potent.

No allergies, so I have no need for Zyrtec which is an anti-histamine. Antihistamine is known to reduce the tear volume causing dry eyes. Now there is no antihistamine in my system. Tear volume returned to normal. My dry eyes are now not dry anymore. They are well lubricated. I think this is the main reason my problem of dry eyes went away like dust in the wind, being free of the anti-histamine Zyrtec? Or are there other reasons too like lowering inflammation avoiding damages to the tear ducts? It is quite possible. But I have the antihistamine to blame now.

Yet in most autoimmune disease in which the immune system is attacking everything in the body including tear ducts, dry eyes is common in those autoimmune diseases like RA. When RA is successfully treated, the dry-eyes go away.

To Sum up -

My dry-eyes resolved as the immune system regained its function, and stopped attacking the tear ducts, just like other autoimmune diseases as in Sjogren's Syndrome, and Rheumatoid Arthritis which commonly have dry-eyes as one of the problems. When the diseases are treated into remission, the dry-eyes disappeared. Functional Medicine physicians have thousands of patients treated like that. And of course, those patients have to be careful to avoid the bad foods that they are sensitive to while the same foods may not be sensitive for other people.

Chapter Sixteen - Why! I was startled and shocked by sudden stereo vision

I was stunned for a few seconds because in my medical learning, this cannot happen. It never occurred in my mind that the herbal supplements could have done this for me.

Try asking a physician educated in the US like me what is the use of pumpkin seed oil. I would be stunned and would be unable to answer, because it involved herbal medicine. I did not learn herbal medicine in medical school.

Unlike European physicians, they have to pass a section on herbal medicine to pass the medical board examination for a license to practice, not in US, though it is for the rest of the world.

Of course, now I have learned enough herbal medicine for my own use. I could tell you that when my urine is slow and weak because of a big prostate (Benign Prostatic Hypertrophy), the pumpkin seed oil could make the flow strong like a wide open faucet, because the pumpkin seed oil can shrink the size of the big prostate. That is awesome and powerful information.

How I wish Herbal Medicine was part of my medical education. Physicians in the rest of the world are using both herbs and traditional medications. But one specialty group of doctors in USA knows herbs are useful for their patients while conventional medications cannot, for some particular diseases.

Eye doctors in the US know some useful herbs

Sir Francis Bacon said it right, "Knowledge is power". Do American physicians want this power of the herbs? The answer is probably a resounding yes. There is no doubt the eye-doctors in the United States have enjoyed this power a little bit. They knew what can slow down age-related macular degeneration (AMD) and cataract, or improve visual sharpness. They have a few supplements at their choice besides traditional medications. Those choices were offered to them from two big golden studies. These are Lutein, Zeaxanthine, vitamins C, E, and minerals zinc, and copper. These were proven in studies to help slow down AMD, cataract, or reverse them. Also they can sharpen vision. These supplements are all anti-oxidants.

When light strikes the eyes (at the retina), a lot of oxidants are generated to burn the neighboring tissues. But the eyes have high concentrations of anti-oxidants (made by our bodies) stored there to neutralize the oxidants. The above external supplements of Lutein and Ziaxanthine are the same anti-oxidants made by the body that got concentrated in the eyes too. But the natural ones can become low. Those supplements come in handy to neutralize the oxidants. How do we know these supplements help?

Supplements come to help patients when traditional medicine cannot slow down the progression of AMD

Two big studies called Age-Related Eye Disease Study 1 and 2 (AREDS I, & II) have shown that those supplements can help to slow down AMD, cataract or reverse them. They may also improve vision sharpness. It seems that no traditional medications have been found yet to slow down AMD.

The AREDS-2, the newer study, uses the supplements as follows:
Lutein-10 mg, Zeaxanthine -2mg, Omega-3 -1000mg, vitamin C–500 mg, vitamin E-400 IU (international units), Copper-2 mg. Zn 80 or 25 mg. In the study, rare side effects were found to be back pain, bruising under the skin (increased chance of bleeding), diarrhea, dizziness, weakness and joint pain.

Here a caution is important. High dose vitamin E at more than 400 IU daily for a long time in terms of years, was found in golden studies to cause increased chance of prostate cancer, and increased hemorrhagic (bleeding) strokes. I take vitamin E only a few times per week and at a lower dose.

All of a sudden, I saw stereo vision

Now please steer away from academics and allow me to get to the lighter part of this chapter. This was about how suddenly I was surprised by a new look of the country side USA. To start with, let me compare Chinese paintings to Western paintings. I enjoyed looking at beautiful Chinese paintings of elegant looking mountains as I was growing up. But they looked flat. By comparison, Western paintings of the countryside usually have foreground and background, appearing in a stereo manner. I love those pictures too.

Most of my adult life while I am driving, the views outside the car was like a Chinese painting. It looked flat, rushing backwards at speed limit. I never got a speeding ticket from a police yet. Also, the views I saw while driving never had stood out as stereotypic.

This all changed in the spring of 2019, after a little more than six months' stay in Florida for the winter. I was driving back to New York along I-95N in order to get back to Long Island New York so I can spoil the three little grandchildren in NY. I have been driving North for years every Spring.

But this time, the familiar views outside the car window were so different. The trees near me stood out as the foreground, with the background forest standing way back. Gee, that is stereo, like a Western painting. That I saw for the first time. I even was able to spot police cars earlier. What a good and practical change.

What happened? I brushed away the possibility of a miracle from a higher being above in the sky. And I remembered I have been taking Lutein and Zeaxanthine for a while along with daily vitamins that contains vitamins E, C, Zn, and Copper and *bilberry*. Now my vision sharpness has become way better, even at night. I can see things more clearly and the stereo vision appeared for the first time, beautiful just like National Geographic videos. Countryside USA has never looked better.

To sum up:

I was taking supplements Lutein and Zeaxanthine, same antioxidants are found in my retina along with Vitamins C and E as well as minerals Zn and copper and herbal supplement *bilberry* for my eye sights. The supplemental vitamins and minerals are mainly supplied by a single multivitamin pill. These supplements have been shown in well-run studies to slow down macular degeneration, and cataract or reverse them. And they improve sharpness of visions too. Lutein and Zeaxanthine comes in one pill usually.

A few months after taking the above supplements, my vision improved so much I could see stereo vision for the first time.

Chapter Seventeen - How I prevented Retinal Bleedings which almost blinded me in the Past

My retinal bleeding was due to diabetes, or rather, due to chronic inflammations. Retina is an inside lining at the back of the eyeballs. There the retina changes light signals into nerve signals. These nerve signals feed into the brain to give us the vision. So we can see the beautiful views of the world.

The retina has a lot of small blood vessels called small arterioles and venules. They are so tiny that they can be very fragile. When light hits the retina, it creates lots of oxidants- -oxidizing damaging molecules. These oxidants can damage the blood vessels in the retina. The damaged blood vessels can bleed and the blood coming out can cause reactions resulting in blindness, if the bleeding happens in the wrong spot of the retina. Though most of the time, when the bleeding stops, the blood can be absorbed back. If the bleeding is so small, they look like a pin head. These are called pin-point hemorrhages (bleedings). Its presence hints at potential bigger bleedings. This is commonly seen in diabetic patients whose blood sugar is high. High level of sugar is inflammatory, because free radicals can come out of the sugar if the sugar level is high. Those free radicals can damage any tissue, including the small blood vessels and make them bleed.

I was found to have pinhead-size bleeding in the retina of the eyes

Almost seven years ago, I was found to have pin-point hemorrhages in my eyes. The retinal specialist knew I am a diabetic, and we both knew this was due to blood sugar not well controlled. But all the time, my blood sugar was pretty well controlled, including the time when the retinal pin-point hemorrhages were seen. I did not understand why it happened at the time. Not until recently after learning facts about systemic chronic inflammation due to eating the wrong foods, then I understood it was due to my chronic inflammation. At that time I had no idea. The inflammation could have hurt the small blood vessels in the eyes resulting in bleedings. Internal inflammation has been proven to heart larger arteries resulting in heart attacks and strokes. It is even easier to get the arterioles and venules in the retinal to be damaged and bleed.

Herbs to the rescue (Can't think about any conventional drugs to help)

But at that time, I was studying herbal medicine to find herbs for fighting cancers. So I looked at various herbs and see what can help with retinal bleeding. *Ginkgo biloba* was the first to be studied. It improves blood flow everywhere including the eyes. I was taking it to quiet down my life-long tinnitus (ringing in the ears). It did lower the decibels of tinnitus. Besides, there was one important benefit. It ended up getting more blood to my private part. Oh, well, that was very welcome. It was described in Chapter Two.

Now can it help with my retinal bleeding? Hell! No. *Ginkgo* was reported in a few cases to cause retinal bleedings (Not pin-point bleedings, but bigger bleedings). I was already taking *Ginkgo biloba* for a few years by then, everyday. So I trimmed it down to 5 days per week. But later on, I realized while I was on it in the past, I never broke out in new retinal hemorrhage anyway. So I continued with *Ginkgo biloba* seven days a week.

I already had studied about *Bilberry* extract. It stabilized retinal vessels reported in studies in PDR for Herbal Medicine. So I started *Bilberry* supplement about 20 mg daily. The first thing I discovered, night driving seemed easier. But I also started taking Lutein and Zeaxanthin. So what made me see better at night is a question. Is it *Bilberry* or the other ones? But it is well publicized that the *bilberry* jam and toast the Royal air-force men took was rumored to let them see their targets better during night air raids in the Second World War. No matter, the question now is whether they can get rid of my pin-point hemorrhages in the retina of my eyes.

Half a year later, in the retinal specialist check up, the pin-point hemorrhages on my retina of the eyes were gone. It never came back for the years in follow up examinations.

How can bilberry be dangerous? People eat it every day

Bilberry supplement is a little dangerous. As per PDR for Herbal Medicine, prolonged use or high dose can cause intoxication.

High dose on animals have been fatal (Eating too much?). So you can see plants can be dangerous. It is no wonder that it worked so well to get rid of my retinal bleeding. It is strong.

In general, taking vitamins or nutrients from whole foods is safer than taking supplements. But even as food, over-eating can be dangerous. People eating too much *Ginkgo biloba* nuts in massive amounts (only need to be 10 nuts or more to be potentially fatal) are known to die of it.

How can I balance the benefit and danger of *bilberry* supplement? If taken long term, it intoxicates

I could not find scientific studies for guidance. So I had to design my regimen of taking *bilberry* supplements half practically, half scientifically. For scientific consideration, long term use is intoxicating means to me that there is some chemicals from *bilberry* that accumulates to affect the central nervous system. The accumulation most likely happened in fatty tissues. It takes long time for drugs to diffuse out of fats. So I need to stop taking it for two days per week for the metabolic chemicals of *bilberry* to dissipate enough before continuing.

On the practical consideration, I don't want to risk bleeding in the eyes, so I will need to continue the *bilberry* supplement on a schedule of two to three days off per week schedule. This scheme worked, I no longer feel slightly intoxicated.

Is it proven effective scientifically? Yes, PDR showed studies proving it improved diabetic retinopathy (includes retinal bleedings) by 77% to 90%. That was why it got rid of my retinal bleedings and helped sharpened my eye-sights.

Interesting study: Can avoid bad foods and eat good foods get rid of retinal pin-head size bleedings? No studies were done

I am not sure if lowering my chronic inflammation alone was able to get rid of the pin-point hemorrhages (bleeding) or not. Since inflammation in the body system is known to weaken blood vessels too, leading to heart attack and strokes (Please see Chapter 10 and 44). Inflammation could easily break the weak small blood vessels. But I only started to tackle my chronic inflammation by avoiding bad inflammatory foods for about 18 months. Bilberry was started 4 years ago, followed by resolution of the pin-point hemorrhages (bleeding). So it was *bilberry* and I had no choice but to continue the *bilberry* supplement. Just to ensure I won't go blind due to bleeding in my retina of the eyes. Lowering inflammation would help by avoiding the inflammatory damages to blood vessels too.

I take *bilberry* in the evening so I can avoid the intoxication with chronic consumption if intoxication is present at night time, I would be sleeping and won't be feeling the slight dizziness.

To sum up -

About two decades ago, a huge area of bleeding occurred to my retina. If it occurred a few millimeters away, it could have blinded me. The eye doc said I was lucky. So when seven years ago, minor bleedings, the pin-point hemorrhages occurred on my retina, I had to hurry to find something to prevent that from developing into a real bleeding. I could not hope to control my sugar in the blood to achieve that, because it was under pretty good control, and so was my hypertension. They shouldn't be the reasons for my retinal bleeding.

As a physician, I know I could not ask for help from standard traditional medications. There was none that could help. Fortunately, I have already studied quite a bit about herbal medicine. I started using *Bilberry* supplement. It worked. The retinal bleeding vanished, and no new ones appeared for the past 5 years. Since I felt slightly intoxicated with taking *bilberry* daily, I started taking it every other day or not taking it in the weekends. The feeling of intoxication stopped.

Once again, I am convinced adding useful herbal medicine learning to medical school curriculum is a good idea. Since there is none in conventional medications that was proven to stop retinal bleeding, now bilberry stopped the pin-point hemorrhages I had. There is eye-sight saving from herbs. It could help millions of diabetic patients to preserve their eye-sights if herbal medicine is a required course in medical schools.

Chapter Eighteen - My gray Hair turned white and curly from a Master Anti-oxidant

This is a case of antioxidant overdose, or the anti-oxidant was just taken superfluously and harmed me more than helped me.

To begin with this Chapter, you would want to know why I started taking a "master" anti-oxidant anyway? The answer was easy. I was following what I thought was a beneficial trend.

Fad diets and beliefs came and went. High dose vitamin C came and gone. High dose vitamin D came and gone. A lot of the fad diets started with New York Times best sellers. A lot of the fad-fashions stayed and became a lasting trend to improve people's lives. Here came another NY Times best seller about ant-oxidant by an honest hard working scientist (19). He spent his long career working on anti-oxidants in his laboratory, made a lot of discoveries. And he became a world-famous Dr Antioxidant.

His book started a popular belief of taking anti-oxidants.

Anti-oxidants neutralize free radicals in our body. Free radicals can injure our tissues in the body. So the more anti-oxidants in our body, the better our body will be protected? This was the on-going thought. This got a lot of people started taking anti-oxidants.

One example I shall not soon forget was the case of four girls poisoned by *Amenita phallodes*, the California Death Cap mushroom, The coded death rate in the book was 3 out of 4 as stated in the book (updated death rate now = 22.4% only, and Silibinin, a milk thistle chemical, may save 100%). As described in the book, when a master antioxidant alpha-lipoic acid (ALA) was used ,it saved three of the four girls while the stated death rate mentioned by the book at that time was 3 out of 4 as described above. So I was impressed with antioxidants right there after reading the book.

The antioxidants I was most impressed with was alpha lipoic acid. I called it a master antioxidant. It can dissolve in fat or water, unlike the other antioxidants that either dissolve in water or fat. Besides, it can reactivate other antioxidants like vitamin E and C. Both vitamins C and E are needed for the health and well-being of the eyes.

So I wanted to give alpha-lipoic acid a trial. I started taking one capsule of 600 mg a day.

Taking antioxidants turned my hair from grey to white

Six months later, my hair was turning whitish-grey, even my wife noticed the hair color change. It was mostly blackish-grey before I started the ALA. At the same time, in the web, people started to complain of various problems arising from taking anti-oxidants. Symptoms like fatigue, loss of appetite, grey hair, memory loss, brain fog, wrinkles etc. Some even labeled it antioxidant stress syndrome.

Biologically not a good idea to take supplements of anti-oxidants

Is it a good idea to take antioxidant supplements? The answer is probably a "No". Why? Here is why, just look at the important functions of oxidants in our body. Then you know it is not a good idea to take supplement antioxidants that circulate all over the body that can wipe out those important functions of the oxidants, especially at high dose.

Most natural anti-oxidants in our body, I suspect, acts locally when required at a particular moment. Like lutein or Zeaxantine, would be locally concentrated in the retina area of the eyes where they are needed to neutralize UV light induced oxidants. By taking anti-oxidants, we are flushing our systems with antioxidants. What is that good for? I don't think it is easy to explain.

Important biological functions of oxidants

Oxidants like hydrogen peroxide kills bacterial as we all know. Oxidants have numerous other important biological functions for our bodies, like making old cells go away by a process called apoptosis, so new cells can replace them. Oxidants help the liver in detoxification by activating P450 system of detoxification. It helps the immune system in an immune function called antigen presentation. In fetus, it stimulates the maturing process (differentiation of the fetus. Women with pregnancy probably should stay away from antioxidant supplements. But eating appropriate amount of antioxidants rich food should be Ok). Oxidants are also a second-messengers for growth signals.

Wiping out oxidants with massive antioxidants is not a good

idea. Take hair growth for example. The growth signal may involve a lot of second messengers. If the alpha lipoic acid got rid of the second messengers for my hair growth, how could my hair grows well. So it started looking grayish-white. I stopped taking alpha lipoic acid, it turned a little more black, as me and my wife could see. But it still was not blacker like it was before.

Gradually, as I started lowering my chronic inflammation by eating good foods, avoiding bad foods, my hair finally turned almost all black.

To sum up -

Oxidants are necessary for a lot of our body's important biological activities. We cannot take antioxidants to interfere with the important functions. Eating whole foods that are high in antioxidants is Ok if not eating a massive amount. That was why my hair turned grey and curly, an unhealthy look, when I was taking a strong antioxidant supplement, alpha lipoic acid (ALA) at the dose labeled in the bottle. I stopped taking ALA. The hair color improved gradually.

Antioxidants are perhaps dangerous to the fetus, because natural oxidants are necessary in fetal development since it promote differentiation of the fetus. So as a precaution in pregnancy, when pregnant, women have to avoid unnecessary drugs, antioxidants probably should be avoided as well.

Chapter Nineteen – A Friend lost 10 lbs with a Lump in the Neck which turned out not to be a Cancer

Losing weight with a lump in the neck means "head and neck cancer" to me as a medical oncologist who specialized in treating cancers. But it turned out to be a good thing. Believe it or not.

It's a long story. But it turned out to be a good thing

This happened to an old friend who is a retired engineer. We got to know each other over the past 35 years, being both frequent swimmers in the same community swimming pool in Long Island, New York. The pool is a 25 meter long pool with six lanes for lap-swimming and a bigger area for water aerobics and another big area for water-slide and other water sprouts for children. It even has a sauna and a steam room, in each of the male and female locker rooms. That is one nice place to be in especially in the cold winters.

Then when I retired and spent the winters in Florida, we found out our old friend John and his wife just happened to live in another apartment building a tranquil pond away (No alligators, That is supposed to be a disappointment in Florida…nothing to watch). So we saw each other now and then. So far, even though getting older and older, no major disaster has struck either of our families yet.

One day, over dinner at home in New York, my wife suddenly said John's wife told her that John lost 10 pounds and has a lump in the neck. This happened after he drove back to New York from Florida, for the summer. With a lymph node in the neck and lost so much weight, an aggressive type of nasopharyngeal (NPC) cancer at once came into my mind. NPC is very common among people in Hong Kong. But patients usually do not lose weight like that. And that type of NPC is very curable with a high percentage of long term survivors.

But a recent new form of NPC in USA is very aggressive and lethal. That type of NPC makes people lose weight and become very weak, especially after chemotherapy.

My wife also told me John was seeing doctors for that problem. I was guessing poor John would be having chemotherapy soon. His hair would be falling out soon. And he would be bed-ridden because of the cancer itself on top of the treatment. My wife and I lost a relative about twenty years ago when he had this aggressive cancer. He was bed-ridden all the time. The relative passed away in about a year after treatment failed to slow down the disease. I wished John luck in my mind. But since they chose not to say anything about it, we respected their wish for privacy and never inquired.

But just thinking about that made my heart sink. John had a good heart. John and his wife took long walks everyday down in Florida. They were keen on keeping a good health. Despite this, he could be dying of a cancer just two years into his retirement. Be weakened so much by cancer and be bound to a hospital bed till the end. What lousy destiny he has, I thought to myself.

One day, in NY, as I entered the sauna in the community swimming pool, I was a little frightened. John seemed alive and well sitting in a corner alone in the sauna, looking very thin, but did not appear sad nor weakened. But he did look a little dark in the dim light of the sauna. I sat down a few spaces from him unconsciously, thinking I must have seen a ghost. But he smiled a little and started talking.

Upon more conversation, he said he was thankful he took my diet advice. That was the advice I gave him half a year ago down in Florida when we met each other during the beach walks. The diet advice I gave was the immune tune-up diet of "Avoid bad foods, eat good foods". Since then, he was eating mainly good vegetable diet with good meats and good fats.

Since he also had an elevated prostate specific antigen (PSA), I also advised him to drink more pomegranate juice (red in color), cook more with turmeric (yellow), and eat more green-leaf vegetables (green). This combination of traffic lights red, yellow and green diet is easy to remember. This "traffic light diet" was recommended to him to see if it would lower his PSA. This diet was found in studies to lower the PSA. Details of his prostate and PSA will be discussed in Chapter 27.

Following the immune tune up diet, he lost five to seven pounds in the half year in Florida. Of course this weight-loss is like everyone who practiced this diet (with exercise or without) would lose about seven pounds without even trying. I told him about the possible unintended weight loss with this healthy diet too in Florida. Ok, this weight was not ten pounds as my wife relayed his wife's words. This is a healthy weight loss, but both my wife and his wife didn't know the reason for the weight loss. They thought some disease made John lose a lot of weight. And with the neck mass, they suspected horrible cancers.

What was the mass on the neck? It turned out to be a thyroid nodule. It was not sure at that time if it was cancer or not. But thyroid nodules are common in 70 years old people. It could be found in more than 70% of the elderly at that age group. His nodule turned out to be non-cancerous after more than a year's follow up with ultrasound.

So a neck mass with 10 pounds weight loss stunned me when John's wife conveyed her worry to my wife and my frightened wife worded it in terms of a very probable bad head and neck cancer. It disturbed my nerve a little. But as a retired medical oncologist, I took cared of cancers patients all my life. The news certainly did not frighten me. But it did sadden me. Though, eventually, it turned out to be a good thing with happy endings – seen alive in the sauna. Why did he lost weight and thanked me?

My friend pursued a Paleo-like/ Mediterranean diet, plus avoiding bad foods, eating good foods. He tuned up his immune system, lost seven pounds. He was seven pounds healthier with a stronger immune system. The stronger immune system would help him preventing cancers. And best of all, the neck mass turned out to be a thyroid nodule and not a cancer lymph node. Right there and then he should have no worries. Lying ahead of him is a bright and joyful retirement for years to come. And he was enjoying the hot toasting air of the sauna, expressing satisfaction in life. And the ghost suddenly turned into a live human being right in front of my eyes.

To sum up:
The fear of cancer frightened people easily as shown in the events in this chapter. But more importantly, the Paleo-like or Mediterranean diet besides making people healthier, it usually brings unintended weight loss which is healthy.

Chapter Twenty – A "cold" for only 3 days for my Wife; for my Son, The "cold" was abolished at the start. Thanks to a combination Supplement

Common Cold got beaten. The Rhino virus killed by its archenemy

For common colds, we all know the conventional treatment is supportive. It runs its course in 5 to 7 days.

While in sunny Florida in April, my wife caught a cold. She started coughing and sneezing. The weather was warm, and flowers had been blooming for a few weeks. So I thought it was allergy. But by the second day, she developed a sore throat. That was not typical of allergy. Then we realized in a warm and sunny place, catching a "cold" was still possible.

Fortunately, stored in the medicine cabinet was a bottle of "Zn Lozenges". So she started sucking on one lozenge every two hours, with a maximum of six per day. According to the label on the bottle, it was safe for her to take since she did not have ragweed allergy or other plant hypersensitivities. And she was not taking BCP (Birth control pill. Its effect weakened by *Echinacea*). At the tender age of 70's, birth control pill is no longer medically necessary. Remember, at this age, 50% of the couples deem sex-life as optional anyway.

By the evening, the sore throat was gone. Then the next day by noon, the common cold was over. By May, we were back in New York.

This time, my son woke up in the morning, feeling a little cold was coming. I advised him to start sucking on the "Zn Lozenges". By mid- day, he was Ok, the common cold never had a chance to start.

What drugs does this Zn lozenge contain?

It is a combination lozenge. Its active ingredients consisted of *Echinacea*, zinc, and vitamin C.

Common cold and vitamin C (100 mg in the combination lozenge, 167% of daily requirement)

Vitamin C is frequently promoted for preventing the common

cold. But in a lot of studies, it failed to prevent any cold. But it does relieve the cold symptoms in some studies. The best reason to include it in the lozenges is perhaps for preventing pneumonia as a result of getting the common cold/flu. This was found in one good study with a group of elderly people. Knowing that when the elderly died of a cold/flu, it frequently is due to the pneumonias as a complication of cold/flu, its inclusion in these lozenges should be a welcome inclusion. Lowering the chances of pneumonia is the same as lowering the chances of death from cold/flu infections for the elderly.

Echinacea can treat common cold and influenza (20 mg in the combination lozenge)

Echinacea is a native plant of USA. It was used for hundreds of years by native American Indians for upper respiratory tract infections. Now it is one of the most popular herbal supplements in the world. It is used for treating the common cold and flu as well as for immune enhancement. Basic scientific studies have shown it kills the flu virus and the cold virus (Rhino virus) and enhance the immune system. But it is ineffective in preventing the common cold or flu.

Precautions written in the labels of the bottle for using *Echinacea* just commonly include warning against grass and ragweed allergies. But besides what is in the label on the bottle, anaphylaxis has been reported. It may also decrease the effectiveness of birth control pills. And it is contraindicated in children less than 13 years old, and women with pregnancy. But for a very rare and small chance, people can get hurt bad, as explained next.

Echinacea is not that harmless; (Never take a herb long term lightly)

But with millions and millions of people using this herb, damages due to people abnormally allergic to it have been seen and reported, no matter how rare. (A lot of people taking it long term for immune enhancement).

Case reports: (Extracted from Memorial Sloan-Kettering Cancer Center website by typing "MSKCC *Echinacea*")

It has been reported to cause problems with bone marrow

depression causing low platelet counts, low white blood cell counts. A 2 years old girl got a kidney failure from it. A young man got TTP from it and had to undergo treatment in the hospital for a month. TTP is thrombotic thrombocytopenic purpura, a very serious disease that carries high mortality if not diagnosed in time and treated in the hospital (Usually in the ICU). *Echinacea* also has been reported to cause bilateral facial palsy and hypereosinophilia also.

That is why herbal literatures always warn of not to take herbs long term. And for *Echinacea,* people with asthma should be cautious about taking it.

Zn is the mineral zinc. It has been shown to prevent the Rhino virus from making copies of itselve (replication). Replication is part of the infection process. Without replication, the infection would stop. The dose of zinc is 23 mg in the combination lozenge. It is 153% of daily requirement.

To sum up:

Echinacea, **Zn, Vitamin C lozenges is a very effective cold/flu fighting drug. Millions and millions of people have used it without problem. But like all other herbal medications, use it with caution. No long term use is without risk. It usually is advisable to avoid giving it to children or pregnant women or people with grass allergies. Echinacea is thought to be very safe, but it does have plenty of idiosyncratic side effects as seen in MSKCC web-site.**

Rare dangers aside, it humbles me more is the fact that our conventional medications can never cure a cold like that.

Chapter Twenty One - How I easily cured my 30-days dry coughing.

Broncospasm

Spasm of the airways of the lungs caused by cold air is very common. It is an allergic reaction to cold air. Airway hypersensitivity is a hereditary trait that runs in my family. But I was never symptomatic to be coughing when I was younger. Some of my family members have it as asthmas when they were very young. It got easier as they grew up, but they never grew out form it.

I cured my yearly cold, but I was still coughing in the winter often

Every early winter for the past seven years, like clock-work, I inevitably caught a mild cold when winter arrived. When the cold was over, I still would be dry coughing daily for a long month before the coughing stopped.

But these two winters, I tuned up my immune system and prevented the yearly cold. So when I started dry coughing, I said to myself, "That is not right. I didn't have the cold, yet I am still coughing like the previous winters". I concluded that I might have developed cold air induced bronchospasm (Bronchus is air tube, going into spasm) without knowing it. And I have been coughing for seven years (after a cold) without diagnosing the problem. Funny enough, when that happened to other people, I diagnosed it right away for the characteristic dry coughing. And I would recommend to those people to use a scar to cover their mouths to breath when going outside in the cold air. This would prevent the bronchus from going into spasm when exposed to cold air. But for seven years, I failed to diagnose it when I actually was coughing my heart out for a whole month because of the cold air that arrived NY in the winter. And the fact that I have developed cold air induced bronchospasm escaped my sharp clinical attention for two years

What did I do to get rid of the cold air induced-coughing from spasm of the airways leading to the lungs?

Then when I was coughing inside the house, the temperature in the house can be adjusted. So I turned the thermostat up two degrees Fahrenheit. Within an hour, my coughing stopped. Only then I suddenly understood, for the past seven winters, I had been coughing for a month after a cold. I could have easily increased the temperature inside the house and avoided all those troublesome bouts of coughing. Was I an idiot? Well, looked like it.

Why do swimmers caught cold more often?

But the cold was mild as only my airway was temporarily weakened after swimming. That is very common with swimmers who frequently have upper airway infections. I think the temporary weakened immune system after strenuous exercise allows the infection to happen. The weakened immune-state after swimming has been proven in studies. Though the weakened immune state only lasts four to six hours. But it was enough to catch the virus somewhere from sick people and develop a cold before the immune system was restored. Last winter, I stayed by myself for four hours after swimming till my immune system recovered. And I also started the Paleo-like/ the Mediterranean diet, and my immune system has been stronger. And I did not get the common cold in the beginning of the winters anymore.

To sum up:

Not all coughing is due to cold/flu. It can be cold air induced allergic coughing or other diseases. When one is outdoors in the cold winter, cover the mouth with a scarf to breathe through it. And make sure it is warm in the house will prevent the cold-air induced bronchospam and coughing.

Chapter Twenty Two – My sun-burn Skin pain gone in Seconds

How I got burned

Fishing is always fun when you can catch fishes. All my life, I had been attempting to catch a fish with a regular fishing rod and reel. But I never caught any fish. That was discouraging, time and time again. But I never gave up, because there was always hope.

That all changed after I retired and started reading fishing books. One of the fishing books had a funny comment. It tells various techniques about fishing. And it concluded that from there on, after reading the book, I should be different than an "idiot holding a fishing rod, standing by the bank clueless". It tells a good timing to catch fish is when the high tide starts going out in inlets etc (Big fishes to be caught at that time as the big fishes finish their feast in the bay)

Indeed, after reading the book, I was a different fisher, though not yet a "king-fisher". I cut the squid into long strips, threw the bait in the direction of the current. So the squid would look like a live tiny fish swaying in the current. This motion of the bait always attracts fishes. From there on, I became a non-idiot fisher, always catching fishes, almost all the time.

One winter day on the east coast of ce Florida in a nice bay, down on the fishing pier of our condo complex, I started fishing in the early afternoon, when the tide was starting to go out. Three hours later, I got more than ten good-size fishes. These were clean water fishes of legal size and number. And I am not a catch-and-release type. I am hungry for the fish protein and the omega-3 fats. These are good foods. They can lower my inflammation in the system. And enough protein and good fat (omega-3) will start fat-burning in my body too. So there is no reason to throw the fish back, unless they are too small. I went up to my apartment happily.

Right when I was changing clothes inside the bath room, I started feeling an intense burning across the back of my neck. No, God did not start punishing me for being a greedy person that caught way too many fishes. But could it be really a punishment? The skin was red and hot with sun-burn across my whole neck in the back. That area was over-exposed to the sun. My long-sleeve shirt failed to cover that spot, though I had rolled the collars up, and the spotty sun-tan lotion failed to protect my poor neck, oh my poor neck, pain too.

What should I use for sun-burn? Quite a bit of stuff in the kitchen besides commercial ones

At that moment, my knowledge of herbal medicine came to life. I could use olive oil to dilute the *Tea Tree* oil. It is said to be effective for skin wounds. But that was too much work. Besides it could be absorbed through the skin and be toxic. Though the diluted amount of *Tea Tree* oil used on the skin topically is usually deemed safe. So are other essential oils like *Chamomile oil, lavender oil, and peppermint oil* diluted, have all be used for minor skin burns. Deep burns are better left for the professionals to be safe.

I looked around the house. I saw the honey in the kitchen. It is a natural antibiotic with lots of proteins for healing. All I needed to do is to smear a thin layer of honey on, let it sit for half an hour to do the cooling and healing job, then washed it off. But just then, I saw the *Aloe vera* growing on the porch. Then I remembered there was a cut leaf of *Aloe vera* in the refrigerator. I got it out, sliced it longitudinally into two flat halves. I ran the wet leaf across the skin in the back of my neck. Ah, it was instant relief! Pain was gone instantly. The good feeling could compare favorably to catching an extra big fish. The gel of the A*loe vera* did its job. I did not have to do more things like washing, cleaning etc. I was careful to use the gel and not the milk which does not work. Then I looked at the mirror. Even the redness was gone. I could never have believed this wonderful plant from nature. The sun-burn disappeared like magic, right away.

Another good choice, properly tested in the lab on animals for burns treatment is *Calendura* cream. But I did not have it at home. This cream is great for baby diaper-rash and costs only a few dollars per tube. If you grow the beautiful *Calendura* flower in the back yard, make a poultice of the flower, it works wonderfully too.

Wait! Ah. Ok. For this one, you may not have to consult a health professional. But you still have to take responsibility for your own decision and action as well as allergic skin reactions, Ok?

Can more serious sun-burn pain use *Aloe vera*?

You bet, though with some reservation. On the same day when I got the sun-burn skin, my wife had been excitedly, happily and busily cleaning fishes on the pier table with a big smile. She got worse sun-burn. The skin was peeling off, and red and painful. *Aloe vera* healed her wound the same, instantly.

An endocrinologist friend of mine, got a sun-burn with peeling skin. And there were some deeper wounds that might have involved the whole layer of her skin. *Aloe vera* stopped the pain instantly. In several days, the wounds healed without a scar. But she is a physician and knew not to get those deep wounds infected. Treating deep wounds as a non-professional is always risky of skin infection with abscesses.

Reservations with *Aloe vera* for deep wounds

So what reservation was there for *Aloe vera* healing wounds? After all, a lot of commercial sunburn products use it as the main ingredient. The reservation is, in real deep wounds, it may delay the wound healing.

There is also a reservation with the use of *Tea Tree* oil. If the sunburn area is too extensive, using a lot of the oil may lead to significant systemic absorption. A few cc absorbed, may put an adult into coma for a few hours.

As you can see, using medicinal herbs is like using conventional drugs. There can be side-effects, drug interactions, or allergic reactions. A safe bet is to consult a health professional knowledgeable with herbs when the wounds are deep.

To sum up -

Aloe vera *is* great for treating mild to moderate sunburn wounds, in fact, it works in other skin wounds too except the real deep skin wounds. There it may delay the healing.

Chapter Twenty Three –I always have to nurse my Back to avoid Backaches

The cause of the backache with a long delay of years for the injury to cause pain

I rode the bicycle to school in Hong Kong for all my high school years. A one-way trip took an hour. It was a bicycle with handle-bars at a racing set-up that requires a lot of movements of the hips, and bending of the back. I always felt tired in the back muscles after going home. No back pain yet in those years.

For the cause of the back pain, studies in the New England Journal of Medicine showed muscle spasm is the cause for almost all back pains. And with each acute back pain attack, it takes around five days to recover by bed rest. No treatments of any kind would change the course.

When was the real bad back pain attack?

I injured my back during high school years, with over-exercises when riding the bike to school daily. X-rays of my back years later when I was a technologist showed arthritis in the hips, especially the left hip. It was the cause for a back pain. But it was not serious pain. There is arthritis in the hip joints. The inflammation there hurts the surrounding muscles. Muscle spasm would cause pain. The real back pain attack that immobilized me did not come till a decade later.

It happened during my second year of the Internal Medicine residency. That morning, I arrived at the hospital parking lot in upper Manhattan. After I parked the car, opened the door and got out of the car in a slightly bent position. As my feet touched the ground and I tried to stand up. An acute back pain that was so sharp, it left me unable to straighten my back to avoid pain. I walked with my back bent into the hospital. My wife came to wheel me on a wheel chair. The orthopedics examined me and sent me home to rest for two weeks. It was the first real back pain in my life, and the worst one. It took seven days to recover from the impossible muscle spasm. X-ray showed a lot of arthritic changes along my left hip. This was the result of the strenuous bike-riding. It injured the hip joint on the left. The chronic inflammation of the hip in turn slowly "burned" the neighboring muscles, making them prone to spasm. Since then, I have to take care of my back like the best nurse on earth. I don't want pain like that anymore.

Why should the injury suffered more than two decades ago caused acute back pain decades later?

It was not that the injury was laying in wait for decades, and all of a sudden attacked me then. It was me, adding a little bit of injury over time, especially during the Internal Medicine Residency training. The work is highly mental. But it also requires a lot of physical work as well. I always went to do resuscitations of patients whose hearts were found not beating. Pushing on the chest to create heart beats for dying patients was hard work on the back, especially several times a day. Of course the work hours were very long in the old days too compared to now. Other physical activities like running around in rapid pace demands a strong physical body too. Finally, the injury caught up with me to give me the back-attack I would never forget.

Methods to keep my back pain at bay

With careful posturing, exercise, using heating methods when the back needs it, and daily self-invented exercises, to support my back when sitting or standing, has kept the back pain from coming back. Never again did I have any severe back pain since that episode. Lowering the inflammation by "eat good foods, avoid bad foods" helped. And recently, back exercise with a resistance machine made my back feel stronger too. But the injury of the years added up, and my weak back is always a source of pain if I ignore it for just a few hours, the back pain would appear to remind me.

I changed my walking posture. That helps a lot

I used to walk with my head slightly dropped, without much hand swings. The weight of the head forward created downward force. My back muscles had to support the bending and became over-worked. So when I first felt the posture of walking made the back uncomfortable on long walks. I changed my posture of walking.

I just extended my chest forward when I am conscious of the slightly head drop, and raised my head straight. The walking was better. Further change in walking posture involved the swing of the arms, and slight turning of my waist from side to side in harmony with the arm swings. The waist movement followed naturally with the gentle arm swings. This walking posture is almost like the Johnny Walker Whisky man walk, just a little less forceful and without the dramatic look nor any whisky. Johnny Walker might be walking very vividly under the natural influence of the spirit. Without the influence of the whisky, I had to remind myself to walk like that a lot of the time. That manner of walking did not become natural until a long time later after I got used to the new walking posture. Whenever I walk like that, the back feels a lot lighter. So I would recommend this walking gait for anyone with back pain. (If they can physically do it). But it is better to talk to a physical therapist for the exact detail.

Swimming helped the hip joints to clean up the waste-products around the sites of arthritis

Swimming in water, the body weight becomes almost weightless. So all the joints are freed of pressure, and can move freely without grinding on each other. These movements of the joints squeeze the waste products from the joints and the cartilages into the circulation. There it is brought away. Among the waste products is lactic acid from energy metabolism and other acidic chemicals from arthritis which is inflammation. Inflammation always has its compliments of acidic chemicals. They need to be clear away. If they remain there, it could burn the joints and the surrounding muscles. And cause annoying mild pain.

The body heat trapped by the back-support belt relieves the pain

My back support belt is a flexible nylon belt. It helps the back in many ways. Its elastic action massages the back muscles as I move around. The massaging helps circulating the blood with the waste products of metabolism out of the joints and muscles.

But if the muscles are cold, the blood vessels become smaller by constriction due to the cold temperature, the circulation will slow down appreciably. Then there would be a slow-down of supply of nutrients and the slow-down of waste disposal. So the muscles have to be kept warm when I have back pain and the temperature is cool or cold.

There another function of the support belt comes in handy. It trapped the body heat, keep the waist warm. Upon warming up, all the blood vessels in the waist open wide. Circulation improves and the massaging action of the belt now is able to augment the circulation. The waste product of metabolism and inflammation due to arthritis that burns tissues of the back got carried away to the joy of the muscles and the joints. They in turn feel good and I feel good. The world even looks different there, well.

Back support belt has a preventive role

The back support belt has another very important use. I put it on before heavy physical activities like vacuum-cleaning the house, or repairing water-fawcetts. It can prevent the back from feeling tired or aching. The Ford Motor Company is the one, I think, encourages the employees to wear back support belt at work. Their accident rate dropped quite a bit. Their backs and minds must be feeling better when wearing the belt for their heavy physical work. That is a kind and clever decision.

I accidentally discovered one most important exercise to relieve back pain (It was an extremely gentle movement compared to "the twist")

This is an exercise I did not find out by experimentation. It just came to me. One nice Sunday in sunny Northern California when I was working as an oncologist, I was studying to update myself on new cancer treatment studies. I was tired and unable to concentrate. So I stood up to study, swinging my arms and rotating my body from side to side in a relaxed, gentle manner. I had a nagging backache after sitting on the chair for a long time. It was bearable. As I kept on swinging and studying at the same time, the movement woke me up and the study became easier, but still I had the mild backache.

After swinging for 100 times or so, suddenly, the backache was gone. It seemed as if the backache suddenly said bye-bye and disappeared. That discovery had, as they say, changed my life for the better. So from then on, whenever I felt the backache, I stood up and swing from side to side 100 times, or more if needed. More than 90% of the time, the back pain went away. And now, each morning after I wake up, I twist gently 100 times or more to wake my mind up and to warm up my back muscles, and relaxing my back muscles too. The day gets better when I do that.

The above four methods can really help relieve the back pain. Two more methods make my back feel lighter and stronger

The lighter part is by lowering the inflammation by avoiding bad foods and eating good foods. (Please see Chapter 1. 39 for details). Since inflammation is a big part of the cause of all chronic disease including arthritis, and now for me, it includes back pain. As I was walking recently, I got the feeling my back seemed to be "lighter". It happened now and then, not all the time.

On the other hand, feeling the back stronger is a persistent feeling. This happened after I started doing back strengthening exercises with the resistance machine. It is one of the equipment in the gymnasium of our condo complex in Florida. The exercise method is printed on the machine. As I did more back-strengthening exercises, I felt my back a lot stronger as days wears on.

Constant vigilance is the most important thing to prevent back pain from coming back

When sitting down, I always need a cushion to support my back so it won't hurt. So vigilance to make sure there is always something to support my back, sitting or standing is necessary. If once I just sit without back-support, I may get the back pain back. So vigilance to make sure is the single most important thing. But how do I support my back when standing. I could not bring a cushion with me all the time, especially when I was still working, and need to make rounds with residents or fellows on the hospital floors. Most of the time, it involved a lot of standing to discuss clinical matters, I made sure I lean on the wall with my shoulder to take the weight so my back did not have to take the weight for couple of hours.

In daily life, if I am walking too long, I make sure I could rest my back every half hour or so by sitting down or leaning on a support somewhere. That has kept me from excruciating back pain for most of my life.

If I am feeling the back pain coming on, I do some back

muscles relaxing exercises, the gentle twisting which I described earlier. To do the gentle twist, I just stand up, turn my body from side to side with my waist gently swaying. A hundred times or two later, I could feel the pain going away. And if the feeling of backache does not disappear, slapping on the elastic back support always helps. So the aching muscles like the body-heat trapped by the back-support. This way, I could get away from even the slightest discomfort in my back.

To sum up:

Back pain is minimal to none if I paid attention to my walking posture, continue my swimming habit, and wear a back support belt when the feeling of the backache was about to come on. The exercise of a simple swing from side to side standing when there is any backache helps. It would stop the pain. Foods have an influence too as well as the back-strengthening exercises from a resistance machine helped the back to feel stronger.

Fellow sufferers, hope these would help.

Chapter Twenty Four – Cracks on the soles of the feet

What was it due to? The cracks on the sole

For the longest time, the soles of my feet thickened and cracked. I thought it was due to diabetes (DM-2) I have. But in diabetics, the blood circulation has to be real bad before the skin thickened and cracks opened. My DM sugar has been in fair control all my life. The circulation in my feet was always good. I could always feel my pedal pulse (pulse felt in the middle of the top of the feet) was always strong. It was not poor circulation that caused the thick skin on the soles and cracks to open up.

It took the learning of herbal medicine and healthy-lifestyle again to solve the puzzle.

Oregano oil gave the answer and got rid of the thick skin and cracks

One day, my right sole of the feet cracked open. It was dry and not painful. Cracks had showed up now and then on soles of the feet for as long as I could remember. I thought it was due to diabetes, though something was not quite right.

The cracks used to be an inch long or less, and 1/8 inch deep. They went away in a week or so. But this time, it was two inches long and ¼ inch deep. It looked terrible. At that time, I had some knowledge of the use of some essential oils. Essential oils from aromatic spices are strongly anti-bacterial, anti-fungal, and anti-viral. Yes these are from cooking spices. But it takes about 50 - 100 pounds to produce a bottle of the essential oil. Their power is very strong. The crack this time was long and deep. I got to sterilize it and not wait for it to go away.

So I tested a touch of *Oregano* oil on the crack to see if it burned me or not. *Oregano* oil is very strong. It would burn if the crack had no intact skin below it. It didn't burn. So I wetted the whole crack with *Oregano* oil and fell asleep soon. In the next morning when I woke up, the crack was gone! Yes, it was really gone, really all gone, vanished without a trace. The skin became intact. I couldn't see which part of the sole-skin had the crack last night. Another eye-opener this healing of the crack by *Oregano* oil is. My skin healed overnight. So my circulation had to be alright. If the circulation was poor, it may not even heal at all. So what caused my thick skin and cracks? It was the dust mites eating the dead skins and creating cracks.

The herbal oil gave the healing, stopped any more cracks on the sole.

So the healing of the crack overnight was due to two things: kill the dust mites, and let the skin heal. First part of the healing was the killing of dust-mites from the crack. They eat dead skins or the top layer of old skin cells called squamous (flat) cells. These cells are there to be shed off constantly. They are dandruff and skin flakes. These are favorite foods for the dust mites. When the dust mites were killed by the *Oregano* oil, the skin healed.

So I did a change of lifestyle and the cracks never came back. The lifestyle that invited the cracks in the past was my walking bare-footed at home. This put the soles of my feet in full contact with the dust mites. They adhere to the soles and had a feast because the thickened skin was layers and layers of fast growing flat cells. How come that happened, the thickened skin? Walking bare-footed requires the skin to be thick, so the skin became thick.

The lifestyle change was simple but 100% effective. I started wearing slippers in the house all the time. And I cleaned my soles daily when taking a shower. So no more dust-mites to nip at my soles, no more cracks anymore, and the skin became normal and not thick.

The ¼ inch thick skin was like psoriasis. It was gradually going away

In psoriasis the patch of surface skin grows fast. They are supposed to be shed off, but don't. So a thickened patch of pink skin appeared. It is an autoimmune-disease, the dysfunctional immune system makes the flat skin cells grow fast and not shed off. This was the same process on the soles of my feet, on my knee caps. They are patches of thickened skin that comes and goes, but now refuse to be shed off.

Finally, after I restored my immune system to be normal (Please see Chapter One), the thickened and rough looking sole skin became normal looking, leaving me with a healthy looking skin with normal thickness. The knee patches of thickened skin (psoriasis) on my knees went away also. The next chapter will described this psoriasis in more details.

To sum up:

The cracks in the soles of my feet were caused by dust mites feeding on the dead thickened skin. The cracks never occurred again after I started wearing slippers in the house. The slippers isolate my soles of the feet from the dust mites. Since I was wearing slippers, there was no need for a thick skin on the sole. The thickness went way down, but still a little thickened and looked unhealthy.

It all became normally thin as I restored my immune system as described in Chapter One, mainly by eating "good foods and avoiding bad foods".

Chapter Twenty Five – My ugly "Psoriasis" on my Knees finally gone

My dark patches of psoriasis on the front of my knees never bothered me. Because they were on the skin over my knee caps, covered by my long pants. They were larger than the diameter of a golf ball at times, sometimes larger.

They did not bother me but it did scare a friend in the swimming pool. He was startled by the black patches on my knee caps. I guessed skin cancer like malignant melanoma could look like that to the layman. Seeing me being calm and cool, knowing I was a cancer specialist, he calmed himself down pretty soon. It still did not bother me. I had gotten use to its presence. It did not itch, nor bleed. It was just two thick dark patches right on my knee caps. They were just there most of the time, though sometimes they went away.

Psoriasis could grow thick very fast, usually when I had more trouble with my irritable bowel syndrome and feeling a constant urgency as a result. It was bad when I was young. My wife used to shave it off with sharp scalpels. But they would grow back slowly.

Psoriasis is not a cancer. It is just an annoying disease, when it happens in an obvious site like the face or elbow. In cancer-study knowledge, I remembered psoriasis people have been associated with cancers inside the body. But in the old days, nobody knew why. Psoriasis is also associated with other chronic diseases like diabetes, asthma, strokes and heart attacks, diseases now we know are caused by inflammation in the body. And psoriasis is related to chronic inflammation also. So if the inflammation in my body goes way down, psoriasis usually disappears too.

What did I do to make psoriasis go away? By the time I studied herbal medicine, I saw examples of herbal drugs putting on the lesion of the skin frequently make them go away. So I put undiluted *Oregano* oil on the patches of psoriasis. Nothing happened the day I put the herbal oil on. I forgot about it but in a week, the whole patch of psoriasis peeled off when I was taking a shower. The underlying skin was never so normal looking before. But slowly, it grew right back. *Aloe vera* was effective in a study to get rid of the psoriasis when smeared on it topically with the fresh *Aloe* juice from the leaf (not the milk). Once when the psoriasis was very thin, I happened to use the *Aloe vera* for sunburn, and I smeared it on my right knee too which did not have sunburn, but it had a thin psoriasis patch right on the knee cap. The next day, I saw a normal looking skin in its place. That is definitely another eye-opener to an old doc who has seen a lot of things. Was the fast healing of the skin a shock? Yes, close to it.

The real cure gradually happened as I restored my immune system by healing the gut by "Avoiding bad foods, eating good foods". (See chapter 39). Chapter One described the "self treatment" to restore the immune system very well also. Now the skin on my right knee is completely normal. The skin on my left knee, where the psoriasis was more persistent in the past, the skin is almost normal.

Do I believe in the power of eating "good foods, avoiding bad foods" or not? You tell me. It even healed my life-long psoriasis. The almighty herbs only got it off temporarily. The most comforting thought in this case is: If the psoriasis is gone, gone would be the risk of internal cancers associated with psoriasis classically.

To sum up -

Psoriasis is due to chronic inflammation inside the body, like other chronic diseases as asthma, irritable bowel syndrome, allergy, arthritis, strokes, heart attacks and cancers.

Chronic inflammation is due to deranged immune system secreting huge amount of inflammatory chemicals, fighting too many foreign objects all the time. The foreign objects get into the body through the leaky guts. Leaky guts happened when we eat the wrong foods that we are allergic to, especially gluten which 80% of us are allergic to it to some degree.

Avoiding those foods, the leaky gut becomes tight. The immune system is restored. Inflammation due to the deranged immune system goes away. Diseases associated with chronic inflammation either go away or have a very low chance of happening again. Psoriasis is cured as long as I am careful with the foods.

The herbal medical drugs that helped control psoriasis were *Aloe vera*, and *Oregano* oil in my experience.

Chapter Twenty Six – Insect Bites and Herbs Miracles and global epidemic implications

Starting this note, I wonder if you know insects are afraid of flying near aromatic plants. They won't fly around trees like *Eucalyptus* trees or *Rosemary* herbs. Those aromatic plants are like a real hell to them. They may get killed if they come very near those plants and stay for a while. If you like the outdoors, you really don't mind the insects going to hell, at least those insects that enjoy biting you.

How I discovered aromatic oil can repel mosquitoes

One evening, I took the garbage can out from the side of the house to the side of the road for pick up the next morning. I got a mosquito-bite within a minute. It was very itchy.

I went in the house, put on *Tea Tree* oil diluted with olive oil (1:1 dilution) on to the mosquito bite-site. The itching stopped almost right away with a sharp light stinging feeling. I was overjoyed because the stinging feeling told me one thing. The bacteria or virus or other microorganisms were injected under my skin by the mosquito. Then they were burned dead. Those bacteria and virus were injected under my skin after the mosquito sucked my blood. I used quite a bit of *Tea Tree* oil. So I was full of the smell of *Tea Tree* oil.

Later that evening, I went out to the same spot again, still with a lot of *Tea Tree* scent in me. I sat on the bench right where I was bitten. I sat for thirty-minutes, with wind blowing in my face, carrying the scent of the *Tea Tree* oil into where the mosquitoes were hiding. I did not know if that drove them away or not. But one thing I did know, I did not get any bites anymore. Only when I went back to the house then did I realized, the *Tea Tree* oil was repelling the mosquito away. The smell of the aromatic essential oil must have frightened them to death. And then I remembered reading something like that in a small herbal book. People generally use *Eucalyptus* oil for insect repelling. But it looks like *Tea Tree* oil can repel the insects too. (*Eucalyptus* oil is what people use to disinfect linens contaminated with bed-bugs, 99% effective at a hundred times dilution with water).

Tea Tree oil stops mosquito-bite itchiness pretty good. And it repels mosquito down-wind of it. But is this the miracle I meant in the title of this chapter? No. It was another essential oil and another tiny critter-bite. This tiny creature was a fly, the size of a pencil tip. It is mostly transparent. So people who got bitten never saw it coming till the biting happens. Then they know they are bitten, because the biting is very painful. These tiny flies, called *ceratopogonidae* are aptly called by a more common name "No-see-um". It means you never see them before the painful bite. The biting brings bacteria, virus, worms, or protozoans that can cause serious diseases in animals and humans.

The first miracle of herbs I witnessed (On my wife's toes no less)

Few years ago, my wife and I were in a sailboat in a quiet marina in North Carolina. It was in the middle of the night. My wife let out a low cry, and her hand was pointing to her toes. The scream was typical of a bite by the "No-see-ums". It is a very painful bite. But this bite brought more than pain. In a minute, a thumb-nail size swelling rose from her second toe, accompanied by intense itching.

The swelling was very rapid. It seemed to increase in size by the minute. Before we could imagine, it grew up to the size of a small chestnut. We did not have cortisone cream that might decrease the swelling in hours or even days. But cortisone does not do much to the intense itching nor would it kill the microorganisms the flies injected. But we did have a bottle of *Oregano* oil, given to us by a seasoned old sailor. He used it for toothache, fever, cold, and for everything when it is properly diluted with olive oil. I had no olive oil, so I diluted the *Oregano* oil in 1:3 dilutions with water. I applied it to the bite wound, which had become one big blister. The itching stopped, but the thumbnail-size blister remained.

We forgot about the blister for about five minutes. Then my wife gave another surprised scream. She once again pointed to her toe. I looked down as an experienced physician would, with careful observation. When I looked at my wife's toes, I almost fainted. Right in front of my eyes, the thumbnail-size blister was gone. The skin looked as if nothing had happened. Gone with it was the virus or fungus or worms etc. One of them caused the rapid swelling, whether it was bacteria, fungus or virus. These agents could have brought my wife some serious illness. Just like mosquito bites bringing *West Nile* virus, ticks bringing Lyme disease. Whatever diseases they could bring, now seemed gone. With the viruses, bacteria, or protozoan, totally gone, probably killed by the diluted *Oregano* oil. Isn't it a miracle?

Oregano oil does not stop the itchiness of mosquito bites, but *Tea Tree* oil does stop mosquito-bite itchiness very well, in my experience. But I am almost sure diluted *Oregano* oil can kill the bugs that potentially can cause deaths to the persons that got bitten. This happened in mosquito bites associated diseases like yellow fever, encephalitis (brain infection), West Nile virus diseases (usually not death but lots of trouble) and others. All aromatic essential oils like *Tea Tree*, *Oregano*, *clove*, *peppermint*, and *Eucalyptus* oils are capable of killing bacteria, fungus, virus, and others by topical application.

One woman's poison is her man's delight (I twisted an idiom a little for the title. And *Oregano* oil can really flatten the swellings from midges bites – what does it mean? To save the world?)

Just this morning, February 11, 2020 (A month later, "lock-down" was advised by the government due to Respiratory virus pandemic), my wife and I had an early morning walk three blocks away to a supermarket. This happened in our winter residency in a resort town in Central Florida. We walked along a tree-lined path with beautiful lawns and shrubs. My wife's black beautiful blouse was see-through at the upper shoulders, pretty elegant looking. As we walked, she felt painful bites where the see-through part was. It was itchy. So itchy I had to scratch it a little for her to sooth it. By the time we got home, I examined her shoulders carefully like a working physician. There were 4 patches of swelling the sizes of fingers and thumbs. Those swelling were 1.5 mm raised with edema fluid. Those were typical "no-see-ums" bites from the mangroves flanking our condo buildings where we live in Florida. The flies had their blood-meals and left some ugly microorganisms under my wife's skin causing the swellings. They are like poisons to my wife. How come it is my delight? Am I ugly?

Oregano oil killed the organisms injected by the midges?

So half an hour later after we arrived home, we calmly put on *Oregano* oils on those patches of bites. In 10 minutes, I looked again, the 4 swellings were all gone. But underneath the normal-looking skin where the blisters were, I could feel lumps under the skin in the previous location of the bubbles, one lump for each bubble. These lumps reminded me of calcified lymphatic nodules when infectious organisms got walled off. But perhaps they were just allergic lumps here? Gone was the itching too.

So the "no-see-ums" are like poison to my wife, but it was a proud delight for me to realize that my wife's suffering was rapidly ended. Just imagine too the suffering of "hell-fire" burning pain that comes after herpes zoster (Shingles) skin healed. And the burning pain can linger on for months. But now the shingles can be rapidly ended too by applying *Tea Tree* oil at the rash stage for my wife as I mentioned in chapter 6. That killed the shingle right there and spared my wife of the post herpetic pain which is "hell-fire" like. That again was my pride.

Imagine one day, every year, millions of people all over the world will not suffer from shingle's lingering burning pain anymore. That is the delight of having an open mind to learn herbal medicine and rip its wonderful benefits for mankind. That is an immense feeling of delight when millions of people can be free of the "hell-fire" pain that could last for months. Could the *Oregano* oil killing the microorganism injected by the flies teach us something?

Global implications of possible fending-off many insect-bite related epidemics

The *Oregano* oil flattened the raised swelling from the midges (No-see-um) bite right away. It could mean the anti-inflammatory power of the *Oregano* oil got rid of the inflammatory immune-reaction that caused the swelling. But I doubt this as Prednisone can do the same, but in hours or days. Now this was immediate. So it is more likely it killed all the microorganisms injected by the fly and the dead microorganisms no longer elicit the immune-fighting that caused the swelling. The dead microorganisms got walled off and those were the lumps I felt under the skin where the swellings were on my wife's shoulders. This is more probable.

The answer to whether the essential oils can kill microorganisms is easy to find out by studies. Anyone?

If this is the case, then, we can get rid of one fever epidemic from the flies (No-see-um) in South America that involved hundreds of thousands of people. The midges inject an arbovirus that caused fever epidemics. Thousands of immune compromised people died of this infection from the midge-bites. This is called Oropouche Fever. One such epidemic happened in Brazilian Amazon in 1978 to 1980. Finally, 263,000 cases were reported. The midges can also inject filarial parasites too.

So it is possible if *Oregano* oil is available, and killed the microorganisms after the bites, then there would be no epidemic of Orov Fever and no parasitic diseases. Similarly, the use of the appropriate essential oils for different insect bites can prevent other insect-born or tick-born diseases. So we can avoid Lymes Disease, West Nile virus infections or even Yellow fever and other equally terrible epidemics.

There are dozens of essential oils that are very anti-bacterial, anti-viral, anti-protozoan, anti-fungal. They are cheap enough and can be put into small vials with eye-drop sprouts, and caps. If such vials are available when we got bitten outdoors, and apply them immediately, all kinds of diseases can be prevented. And thus epidemics can be prevented. All we have to do is to try to see which essential oil kills which virus or other microorganisms for different epidemics. Then the cure can be bottled into vials.

Should this be the goal for the scientists/governments, health organizations/Big Pharma/World Health Organization's to strive together to eradicate epidemics the easy way?

To sum up:

I witnessed a first miraculous herbal-cure of a blister gone in five minutes on my wife's second toe ten years ago. Then a second time around for more blisters by "no-see-ums" eradicated right away with *Oregano* oil again. As an American-trained physician, I think that was a miracle by the *Oregano* oil. It may not be that miraculous to any physicians trained outside of the United States. They all know the use of herbs as they are required to pass the section on herbal medicine to be licensed to practice.

Yet another potential global miracle can happen if all mosquito-bites or other insect-bites could be sterilized by the appropriate essential oils applied topically right after the bites.

Then there will be no Yellow Fever (Yes, there is the expensive vaccine), Japanese Encephalitis, West Nile disease and (no) other deadly insect-bite related diseases, some cause epidemics. So a possible global implication would be to use essential oils after mosquito bites and fly bites or tick bites. Then all those nasty viruses or organisms can all be killed and not be able to cause all these terrible insect-bites associated epidemics.

A lot of work maybe involved to test and see if this is really the case. If it is, it also is a lot of efforts to achieve the goals of insect-bite epidemic prevention and making the essential oils bottled into small vials for people to use.

But in the first place, has it been done? If not, it is at least worthwhile to start looking into it. Millions of lives may be saved, as well as billions of dollars for the care of the debilitated patients like, for example, in Lyme's Disease.

Chapter Twenty Seven – How a Friend's elevated PSA went down on Diet and Exercise only

PSA and prostate problems

PSA stands for prostate specific antigen. It is secreted by the prostate grand. Blood test can detect it at very low level like at 1 or 2 ng/ml normally. If the PSA is above 4ng/ml, classically, prostate cancer is a possibility. Recent studies even lowered down the PSA level to 2.5 ng/ml as the cut-off point. A level greater than 2.5 ng/ml would lead to the suspicion of prostate cancers.

For decades, prostate cancer is considered a slow growing cancer. Most elderly who have it would die of other medical reasons or dying of old age rather than the prostate cancer. Though rarely younger patients in their 40's and 50's with prostate cancers could have an aggressive course and die from it.

An old friend got a PSA of higher than 4 ng/ml

This is a healthy old friend I got to know from the community swimming pool in Long Island, New York. I saw him in the pool now and then for about 35 years.

The pool is a 25 meter long pool with six lanes for lap-swimming and a bigger area for water aerobics and another big area for water-slide and other water sprouts for children. It even has a sauna and a steam room each in the male or female locker rooms. That is one nice place to be in especially in the cold winters.

With PSA above 4.0 ng/ml, most patients would choose to be followed with "watchful waiting", even if it is cancer. It involves blood tests for PSA periodically every few months to six months or a year. This is chosen by most people because the prostate cancers in the old days were very slow-growing.

This high percentage of slow-growing prostate cancers may be dropping because people are getting more overweight. Obesity increases the whole body inflammation. Recent studies have started to show the higher the inflammation level, the higher the PSA may rise. Though, historically, prostate cancer is the least associated with inflammation, unlike lung and colon cancers. But new studies showed prostate cancer is affected by inflammation in the body as well. Even with a rather insensitive test for inflammation like CPR, the PSA was shown to be higher when the inflammation is higher.

When the systemic (whole body) inflammation went down, the PSA went down

Since my friend had an elevated prostate specific antigen (PSA) of 4.3 ng/ml, though was followed with his own doctor, as a friend, I advised him to drink more pomegranate juice (red in color), cook more with turmeric (yellow), and eat more green-leaf vegetables (green). This combination of red, yellow and green diet is just like the red, yellow and green traffic lights, making it easy to remember. This "traffic light diet" was recommended to him to see if it would lower his PSA. This diet combination of red, yellow and green was studied and was able to lower the PSA. This diet is characteristic of diets that lower inflammation in the body.

But other life-style changes or foods can also lower systemic inflammation too. This is the "avoid bad foods, choose good foods" diet. (See Chapter 39). But the diet that was originally found to lower inflammation are Paleo diet or Mediterranean diet.

To say briefly what the main theme of the Paleo/Mediterranean diets is simple-avoid inflammatory foods and eat anti-inflammatory foods.

Eat foods that the Old Stone Age (Paleolithic) people ate or eat food like the EU people eat. That also means we should stay away from *milk, wheat, sugar and salt. Eat good protein, good fats, and good carbohydrates.*

Good proteins are the meats that are low in saturated fat, white meats like chicken, fish, turkey, lean meats like grass-fed beef, free range chicken meat and eggs and other sea-foods.

Good carbohydrates are the ones that are not starchy. An example of starchy food is potato.

Good fats include fatty fish, olive oil, olive, seeds and nuts, avocado, and dark chocolates, duck fats, coconut oils. The underlying sciences will be explained in Part Two under "New Sciences" in the chapter of "Good foods, Bad foods" in chapter 39.

My old friend was keen on trying to get his PSA down. He

really avoided sugar and milk and cheese most of the time, but not bread (gluten in wheat). He started eating a lot of non-starchy vegetables along with good proteins and good fats. This ought to lower his whole-body inflammation way down. Did it lower the PSA?

Yes, his PSA was 4.5 ng/ml when first found. Repeated a year later, it was 4.2 ng/ml. These levels showed stability. PSA being stable over a year meant it was probably not cancerous. Since he really avoided sugar, and milk and cheese and started eating a lot of non-starchy vegetables. The PSA finally went down to 2.38 ng/ml in six months. He still was eating a piece of toast every morning. So he was not very sensitive to the gluten contained in the bread.

This is good news, because if this is prostate cancer, the PSA will probably not go down like that. It brought great relief to an old friend. He also lost his belly fat without even trying.

I am sure this has made him a true believer in "avoiding bad foods, and chose good foods and eating a lot of non-starchy vegetables.

To sum up:

Diets that lower systemic (whole body) inflammation are able to lower PSA and get rid of a belly fat as shown in one of my old friends. Of course, his raised PSA was not from cancer as long as we can see with modern medical detection. But was it cancer related raised PSA in his case? He refused biopsy, so it is impossible to say. By the fact that the PSA went down implies a non-cancer situation.

It would be nice if initial prostate cancer can be controlled with lowering inflammation. But for now, this possibility sound more like a dream then being real. But no one knows for sure. My friend knew PSA has to be followed with his doctor in the future.

Chapter Twenty Eight – Easy cures for fungus, but not easy for cancers. Yet the key is: What is the cause?

The first fungus infection happened when I was in high school in Hong Kong. The skin in my whole inguinal area (groin) became intensely itchy, red, rough and inflamed. The area was always moist and wet with skin secretions in a warm and moist city like Hong Kong.

My first attempt at self-cure: What a miserable failure!

So even in my high school years, I was keen on playing doctors. I like reading health information in newspapers. Once I read in a newspaper, using corn-starch could dry up the fungus, and made the itchiness disappear. Just like some misinformation in the internet nowadays giving out well-intended but untrue advice. This one advice was terribly wrong.

The corn-starch was in the kitchen handily. So I put it right on my wet groins. In ten minutes, my groin was not itching anymore. It was burning hot almost like a "hell-fire"! Well, not every experiment I did succeeded. That was one blatant example. I hurried to the bathroom and washed the corn-starch off thoroughly. What happened? The corn-starch was a devil-given food for the fungus. They grew happily and rapidly like wild-fire and attacked me like mad. Was that lesson well-learned? Nope! Nothing could ever extinguish my spirit of experimentation, ever.

But I did the right thing next. I went to the doctor who gave me Lamisil. It was in a pill form. I took it religiously for six weeks. But the jock itch wouldn't leave my right groin. I figured it was time for another experiment to cure this jock itch.

Success came way too easy

Finally, I went to the library to read health books about jock itch. I found one basic secret for the fungal growth. They thrived in moist and warm environment, and thrived they did in my warm and moist body areas. So I just started wearing my pants without the cotton under-pant. Right away, my groins were feeling cool and calm. It became well aerated. Just like magic, the itchiness went right away. As for the fungus, it disappeared in a couple of weeks or so. Ha! This experiment was a great success.

The most precious knowledge I ever learned

Curing the fungus at its cause, I learned a lesson for life: To treat a disease well, I have to find the cause and get rid of the cause. In this case, the real cause the moist and warm environment that invited the fungus to grow. This had great influence on my whole life. I saw the horror of cancer done to people and their families. So what was the cause of cancer? I searched hard and long, after 53 years, I found it. But before I revealed the total package to fight cancer, let me add another case of (tinea) fungus (so called ring worm) treatment success with something you would never have guessed. This everybody has at home. And the cure took one night, not six weeks with conventional treatments of the old days. This home remedy is garlic, finely chopped.

This case was 60 years later than the first case. Being warm and moist is the same in Florida. The treatment seemed more sophisticated this time even though it was garlic. My wife had two ring shaped rash on top of two feet. I chopped up the garlic finely, so to make it more powerful. I just mixed a poultice with olive oil, diluting it till it just stings. Then apply the garlic poultice to the ring worms, the size of jumbo eggs, and wrapped it with cloth-bandage to allow aeration.

One night, the tinea pedis was gone. Yes, the "ringworm" was gone in one night. The skin was scalded. So the sophistication called for *Aloe vera* sap. Another few days, only good skin left, no more fungus nor "ringworm". So now let's get back to a more serious topic.

What is the cause of cancer?

That was the question I have been thinking all the time since I worked as a radiation therapy technologist in 1967. So if I wanted to cure cancer, I have to find the cause. That had become my lifelong obsession, and the only goal in my life. Nothing beats a goal of life to do common good. But the answer took me 53 years to come by.

Now it is well-known and commonly accepted cancer starts after the gene mutated. As the gene of a cell is mutated, there is some new antigens (structures) appearing on the surface of the cells expressing itself as "Hey, I'm a foreign object". And the immune surveillance cells will label it for destruction. So if the immune system is normal, it will be potent enough to destroy the new cancer cells. Cancer will only grow if the immune system is dysfunctional.

So the real cause of cancer should be said as due to a dysfunctional immune system, not mutation.

My life-long goal might have been realized

A weaken immune system allows cancer to grow. So the solution of getting rid of cancers is to restore the potent immune-system. It just might be the key in the fight against cancers. So to stop cancer-growth is to remove the cause. And the cause of cancer is the weakened immune system. And now we know a lot more about how to restore the immune potency of ordinary folks. If cancer happens, restoring the immune system can help along with the conventional treatments. Why not? This point was discussed well in Chapter One.

The complete package of helping to fight cancer

And now with the smart life-style against cancer that has been proven to myself. It benefited my patients before I retired, and plus the new leaning of how to restore one's immune system mainly by "Avoiding bad foods, eating only good foods". It becomes the complete set of weapon against cancers. I healed my gut, restored my immune system and got rid of the yearly colds/flu. It most probably should be enough to watch out for cancers that start to appear and get rid of them in the beginning. I think I have realized my lifelong goal of doing the best to fight cancers, by prevention (chapter 51 for more details).

My belief is that if the immune system is restored, cancer can be prevented. So the one thing to do to fight cancer is to restore the immune system to its normal potency to prevent cancer. The contents in chapter one made the statement strongly.

To sum up:

The true cause of the jock itch was due to the moist and warm environment created by the cotton under-pant. I cured my jock itch by ventilating my long pants well without underpants. Sixty years later, garlic cured the foot fungus in one night.

The lesson learned led the way for me to find the true cause of cancer. It may not be the mutation of cells. It might just be a weakened and deranged immune system that let cancers grow.

Chapter Twenty Nine – How I have controlled my Normal Pressure Glaucoma

What is glaucoma?

Glaucoma is the leading cause of blindness world-wide. In the US alone, for people older than 40 years old, there are more than 3 million people went blind because of glaucoma. The problem is: It does not cause pain usually, and the shrinking of the vision happened silently. It could creep up on anybody, and brings blindness. But if it is detected by an eye-doctor (ophthalmologist) in time, it can usually be stopped for most people. And blindness can be prevented.

What is glaucoma? It is a disease in which our vision (so called visual field) shrinks overtime slowly, stealthily. Our visual field is in the shape of a big circle. Glaucoma makes us lose vision at the edge of the circle which shrinks smaller and smaller, till it closes the circle. Closing the circle is blindness. Right? Though the most common form of glaucoma has no symptoms, but people may experience blurred vision or distorted vision during the slow progression of glaucoma. One form of glaucoma may cause severe eye pain. If not treated as emergency, it causes loss of vision rapidly.

What is the real cause of glaucoma?

Most people are familiar with higher ocular (eye) pressure as the cause of glaucoma. But some glaucoma has normal eye pressure. Some glaucoma has low eye pressure. So the common way of equating glaucoma with higher ocular pressure does not mean the cause.

With lots of scientists working on the real causes of glaucoma, there came twelve hypotheses. It's really confusing indeed. One of the causes is thought to be a blood flow problem. In other words, it is a vascular (blood vessel) problem that leaks the flow of eye-water (aqueous humor) leading to building up of pressure. Or the returning route (to the heart) for the eye water slowed down in the veins. Or the vascular problem could be vessel loss (loss of small arteries or veins). And vessel loss could lead to nerve loss. Our vision depends on nerves. Nerves goes, vision goes. The last cause may be more likely.

That is simple and "mechanical". "Mechanical" is the rule in biological processes on molecular biology level.

Is the real cause of glaucoma a vascular problem?

So I set out to ask this question from a 3 to 5-stars eye doctor who is board-certified in the specialty of the retina (one anatomical part of the eye); and also certified in cosmetic surgery. He is David Schlessinger, MD in Long Island NY. Before I could finish the question "What is the cause of glaucoma?" He casually answered, "We think it is a blood flow problem back in medical school". There I got the confirmation from an authoritative professional. The cause of glaucoma is most probably a vascular problem.

My weird presentation of a visual field test result

For glaucoma, the visual field result should show a smaller and smaller circle of vision. But my loss of vision is on the left and right side, not circular. My optic nerve is abnormal but my ocular pressure was always normal for over ten years, so was the visual field results were without any worsening. It was always the same for 10 years. But optic nerve seen abnormal in my case is highly suspicious of glaucoma.

Some herbs I started taking three years ago happened to treat glaucoma

Luck strikes again. I started *ginkgo biloba* and later *bilberry* supplements. Both taken together in a study showed they could slow down glaucoma well. So I was blessed again. I started those herbs for entirely different reasons. But they probably have been helpful in keeping my glaucoma in check by tuning up blood flow, and tuning up blood vessels. I started *ginkgo biloba* for my tinnitus (It helped ED more than tinnitus). Later I started *bilberry* when my vision was bad at night and there was pin-point bleedings in my retina (part of the eyes). They were helpful on both counts. I could see better at night and my pin-point hemorrhages disappeared and never have returned yet.

How did *Ginkgo biloba* help?

The *Ginkgo* trees are living fossils. They existed on earth 270 million years ago, well before the dinosaur era or just at the beginning of the dinosaur era. I could equate *Ginkgo biloba* trees with wilderness because, after Ice-Age, the only surviving forest of *Ginkgo* was found in wilderness location in China, but now they are growing along many streets in one of the most modern city-Manhattan. They were probably chosen to be planted there because it survives in very harsh environment.

Now let's get back to a more pleasant endeavor of books and knowledge. Forget the exciting NYC, it is being locked down for the HEART ATTACK of 2019. The *Ginkgo biloba* helps by increasing blood flow in the body, in the brain for mental things, in the lower legs to help pain on walking (claudication). Last but not the least, it increases blood flow to the eyes in studies too. Also has been studied, it increases blood flow to the penis as well. It achieves the increased flow mainly by dilating blood vessels of small arteries and veins.

Ginkgo biloba dilates small veins in the eye, so the water (aqueous humor) can flow away from the eyes more quickly. It seems to help keeping the eye (ocular) pressure in the right range for people with glaucoma.

Ginkgo biloba taken at high dose can be lethal

It has a chemical called ginkgoside, if accumulated at high level, can cause nausea, vomiting, seizure and rarely, death. Given rare is rare. But there is no lack of reports of people dying after eating too much *Ginkgo* nuts in Asia.

How did *Bilberry* supplement help?

Bilberry stops fragile new small venules and arterioles (small veins and arteries) from being formed (Good for stopping cancer?). Thus it assures only good blood vessels are formed for circulatory needs. This is the basic mechanism of preventing pin-point hemorrhage- by preventing fragile vessels being formed and likely to burst and bleed. This property helps to make new healthy vessels to circulate the water (aqueous humor) away from the eyes in glaucoma.

Bilberry is like blue berry fruit, anything to worry about?

Yes sir. Long term consumption like taking *bilberry* supplement continuously everyday would cause chronic intoxication. It could bring dizziness and staggering gaits. I am taking it to prevent my pin-point bleeding, every other day, still I would have fleeting moments of dizziness on rare occasions that lasted only for split seconds. So I take it in the evening to sleep with the intoxication.

New preventive lifestyles next, it's perhaps the most important to prevent glaucoma by improving blood vessel health

The conventional drugs are just treating the symptoms of higher ocular pressure. The supplements *Bilberry* and *Ginkgo biloba* are treating the cause, i.e. treating the vascular problems. They are more potent than treating the symptoms. But the most important is removing the cause of the vascular problem. It may prevent glaucomas.

The vessels constrict and become fragile because of inflammation, as shown in studies. So if you remove the cause, the inflammation. Glaucoma would not have happened in the first place. The most important treatment for preventing inflammation is to foster a good gut health. The methods to lower inflammation by fostering gut health is to avoid allergic foods (to you), and eat good foods that are anti-inflammatory. The methods are discussed in detail in Chapter 1, 39, and Chapter 42. But this remains a proposed hypothesis that needs studies to confirm.

To sum up:

I have been taking *Bilberry* and *Ginkgo* at recommended dose written on labels on the bottles. Together they have kept my glaucoma damage of my vision not progressing for more than a decade now. But as written in this chapter, there are potential great dangers in taking them. One really needs to be safe to consult a health professional before taking them. *Bilberry* can intoxicate, and overdose on Ginkgo could cause death.

But the most important treatment for glaucoma is to avoid them in the first place. Lowering systemic whole body inflammation would avoid making the veins weak, fragile and constricted. Inflammation even can cause large arteries to be injured and cause strokes and heart attacks (chapter 44).

When the small veins are open, there would not be any build up of eye pressure. Then there would be no glaucoma in the first place. Though for sure as a treatment protocol, this hypothesis still need "golden" studies to prove before anyone can depend on it to treat or prevent glaucoma.

Chapter Thirty - How I cured my Acid Reflux by smart Life-styling alone

Acid reflux is just heart-burns. Avoiding it is better than treating it the conventional way

Heartburn is just nuisance. I was not about to talk about it too long. To begin with, you are tired of hearing and expect me to say, "Stay away from smoking, alcohol, coffee, tea, spicy foods, nuts, tomatoes and the like". So I will not mention about them at all. But I cannot help mentioning a historical national forefather-like figure Benjamin Franklin. He was slightly obese. His being overweight was a healthy kind of overweight. But we have to concentrate on obesity here. The gut specialists of America claimed obesity is #1 cause of acid reflux. The increased abdominal pressure forced the acid up our throats. That's real heart burn. I guess you can feel the pain like some of the 60% of Americans who are overweight.

On the other hand, thanks to Sir Franklin for his bringing attention to Calorie Restriction, which is the same as "to eat 80% full and stop". Eating only 80% full means the stomach is not full, acid would not come up easy. But more importantly, it leads to weight loss. Weight loss is the most efficient way to stop acid reflux for most overweight people. Period.

Unconventional ways of stopping acid reflux pain

Unconventional way #1 is to use bricks to pop up the head of the bed. The head of the bed being just a few inches higher makes a huge difference. When we are sleeping, acid will not flow uphill to burn our throat. Our throats would be spared of the acid burn. I used this method all my life and it worked. I never had heartburn no matter what good fats I eat at dinner.

Unconventional way #2 is something you won't expect. It is to "avoid bad foods and eat good foods (except don't eat a lot of good fats at dinners-moderation is precious)". Avoiding bad inflammation causing foods leads to healing of the gut wall. A non-leaky gut wall shut out millions of foreign objects. No foreign objects in the blood stream, the immune system quiets down. All our system functions run smoothly when that happens. The gut system benefits immediately from a healed gut wall. It regain its good peristalsis (gut contraction waves moving food down). So the active movement of the guts brings food down and out of the stomach. No food in the stomach, no acid secreted. No heartburn ensures.

To sum up:

The conventional ways are to avoid foods that cause high acid secretion and to avoid obesity with a big belly pushing acid up the throat.

The unconventional ways involves popping up the head of the bed so acid cannot flow uphill towards our throats. Also healing the gut wall allows a healthy gut wall to create lovely intestinal waves to bring the foods away from the stomach. No food in the stomach, then there is no acid secretion.

New sciences bring us ways to lower internal inflammation which let the electric wave-like "bowel movement" (peristalsis) to bring food down the intestinal tract away from the stomach, and no food in the stomach, then there is no acid secretion in the stomach to "reflux".

So prevention is my tactic rather than using all those OTC medications.

Chapter Thirty One - How I controlled my horrible Mood-Swings

Mood-Swings led me to quit my first physician-job, or was it depression that failed me?

I have to be honest and say it as it was. I was a radiation therapy training doctor right after medical school graduation in NY. Once, I raised my voice in speaking to a very senior physician, because of a negligible difference of opinion in radiation treatment-planning of a patient. I had seen thousands of treatment plans when I was a radiation therapy technologist. But that was a very rude way to treat my senior.

At that time in my career, I decided to leave radiation therapy as I was still looking to find the cause of cancer. And I also want to learn more research to cure cancer. So I voluntarily stopped radiation therapy training. But nevertheless, it was a failure. But fortunately, I remember the saying, "To fall is human, to rise up again is golden". So life went on, and I had a joyful career in medical oncology rather than radiation oncology, after a few years' worth of pure learning about cancer sciences in a medical college in the evening and later in a cancer research center fulltime. That is all behind me now, for now.

But the real reasons for that failure-event were twofold, besides the desire to continue my goal to look for the cause of cancers, I was also very depressed to see patients not doing well in the radiation therapy department. I just didn't understand why I was so depressed in the radiation department at that time. But now I fully understand.

A deeply-hidden sad-cry in my heart

In 1967, I started taking care of patients with cancers. Saw hundred of them died shortly after I gave radiation treatments to them as a technologist. I developed a sad cry in my heart," Patients with cancers should not die, there ought to be a cure!"

This hidden sad cry has been driving me to find the real cause of cancer, and thus achieve a real cure. It did depress me all my life.

Only when I finally found the true cause of cancers, as I stated in chapter 28, it is due to a deranged immune system which let cancer starts and grow. To restore the immune potency is able to stop cancers at their beginnings.

Since I found the cause of cancer, the hidden sad cry only then surfaced. And it was only then, I realized it. Now I am totally relieved.

Later, after I became a chemotherapy specialist, I was more understanding of why I was depressed at that particular time. Most patients were only sent to have radiation therapy for comfort-treatments (palliation treatment). Treating patients with only months to live were very depressing for me. Anyone could feel the sadness in those patients who know their survival is short, very short.

Now as I learn more about diet and depression. Then I know now the other reason was the typical American diet that caused inflammation in me, and brought with it the mood-swings that I now find it to be a very strange bed-fellow, as I am eating a lot of anti-inflammatory foods and am feeling so mellow as to say to myself, "What mood swings?".

Mood-swings indeed can easily be eliminated out of one's life, so one does not have to feel sorry for some deeds

But mood-swings and loosing tempers like the ones I had while in training in radiation therapy can easily be eliminated. This I learned only in the past two years. How I wish I had known it when I was younger. Then I would not have offended a senior doctor who I respected very much all my life. Fortunately in the past, I only had such bad mood-swings very rarely, might be just once in a blue moon.

How did I get rid of my mood-swings? I honest did not believe I could do it. But all the books written by physicians practicing Functional Medicine say mood-swings can just disappear if you heal your gut, but I was still very skeptical. After all, what has the gut to do with the brain? (It really has everything to do, chapter 40 explains).

But as I avoided the foods I am sensitive to, it happened without me realizing it. My mood became 100% better. Not because I am retired and can just go fishing anytime. There is this good book to write that creates pressure and anxiety like the times of being an oncologist.

Everybody has different food sensitivities, but a lot of people are sensitive to foods brought on by the agricultural revolution and to foods by "cattle farms". Those sensitivities to foods may not cause problems in a lot of people. But a lot of people break out in asthma, sinus problems, lacking energy, and having frequent mood-swings and depressions. And they don't know it is all caused by the wrong foods.

I have some of those problems. So I would benefit from avoiding foods with gluten that include bread, cakes, biscuits and a lot of processed foods that use flour. Also a big item of sensitivity to me is sugar. I have diabetes and could not control blood sugar level well. Enough sugar will raise the blood level high enough so that some sugar would generate free radicals. This brings inflammation and mood-swings and a whole lot of the chronic diseases. The other foods that bring me bad gut health are milk and cheese or other milk products. The resulting high inflammation level will mess up my thought process and mood control. I am so sorry that I never knew that before.

But the worst offender-food for me is the greasy foods in restaurants cooked with trans fats. It guarantees diarrheas in me.

Avoiding bad foods, my mood became mellow before I realized.

There came a whole new world. The new world is tranquil, orderly, peaceful, and pleasant. I became more tolerant of different opinions. I lost the feeling of pride which seems to me now to be unimportant, though it is still a good feeling. So the functional medicine men/women are right. They told the truth because that was what their patients showed them and told them. There are thousands of such patients for each Functional Medicine doc.

Avoiding bad foods brings a whole different world. The new world is like sailing on calm flat seas in constant gentle winds, so called smooth-sailing. The old world was like riding a rough boat on gale force winds. (I don't mind sailing like that except for my wife).

I highly recommend this to anybody. Feeling mellow should be in everybody's life.

To sum up:

Avoiding bad foods and healing the guts as described in this book especially in Chapters 1, and 39, one can bring a peaceful mental status. It's like living in another new peaceful world. Mood-swings, anger and depression are absent or minimal naturally in this new world. Life became more enjoyable for me.

Hopefully it is going to be the same for you.

Chapter Thirty Two – How I improved my Short-term Memory and Mental Acuity

What evaluation methods I used?

I just compared my memory and mental acuity when I was in Hong Kong and shortly after when I am in the United States. I did not use any complicated psychological testing on myself.

When I was in Hong Kong, my mental state was excellent

My thinking process was clear and fast, memory was very good. In fact, when I was still in high school, there was an unofficial IQ test conducted for all the students in the huge meeting hall. I scored an unofficial 167 points. Hong Kong at that time was still a British colony. The test was very valid to me, though I did not get invited to join as a member of the British High IQ club with a 140 points cut-off.

Did I care? No. I cared much more about after school activities, like long hiking, swimming, hiking mountain trails or just playing around. In those days, for me, it was like the song "Mississippi Moon won't you keep on shining on me". "I ain't got no worries, ain't in no hurry at all" as the song goes. Why? Because "playing" is everything!

Diet for top mental performance in Hong Kong

At that time, my diet in the poor family was mainly vegetarian, and the family had no money to buy food for breakfast. I never ate bread, nor drink milk with sweet cereals or ate any eggs. Did I ever feel hungry? Yes, all the time I was hungry, but my personality of forgetting the adversity made me feel life was good. I did not feel the constant hunger at all. So I was so much surprised when my younger brother, at his late 60's, still remembered those mornings of empty stomach during classes.

I guessed I lived like the Paleolithic (Old Stone Age) people, living with constant hunger as part of the normal life. The now popular Paleo diet has the main points of avoiding wheat, milk, and sugar, (but forgetting hunger was part of the "diet" too). The foods avoided are foods that were brought on by the agricultural revolution of planting wheat for food, keeping cows for milk and so on. That happened ten thousand years ago. But our genes for digestion had been fixed millions of years before that, the same genes the Paleolithic people had. These genes evolved for us millions of years in human history before the "recent" agricultural revolution.

So I was eating healthy foods I could easily digest and my mental status was at the tops in Hong Kong.

Diet for compromised mental performance (Different sets of diets gave me different mental status)

Since I came to the United States to start a job in Memorial Sloan Kettering Cancer Center as a radiation therapy technologist, I got a pretty good income, matching medical interns and residents. Ah, food for the American dream became a norm. My diet is consisting of bread, milk and eggs and desserts and fast foods. Ah! This was good American life leading to obesity.

Fortunately working full-time and attending college in the evening in the competitive "pre-med" classes let me used enough energy to avoid obesity. But mental acuity suffered.

But we know a lot of people are sensitive to the "American diet" which is very inflammatory for me. So my mental acuity declined but fortunately was still functional. I did pretty good on this compromised mental performance.

After medical school graduation, I took up cancer care again. With my good heart for the patients who had cancers. My lifestyle-advices enabled the patients to live longer, and had fewer cancer recurrences. Devotion to patients kept my mental acuity up, though not in the tops. Eventually patients even gave me a 5-star rating in return. So my mental status had to be Ok. But I still had mood-swings, mild brain fogs, and only fair recent memory.

The recent memory became good when I learned memory techniques. I made cartoons out of tasks I had to remember to do. The pictures are easier to recall when needed than trying to remember words. But when I was in Hong Kong, I didn't have to do that. Memory came naturally.

Different diets gave me different sets of mental status.

Top mental status of mine returned on

Paleo/Mediterranean diets

My wife used to remind me of the tasks of daily living since we came to the US. My compromised mental status due to fast food diets made me somewhat forgetful. Little things I frequently kept in my mind and not recalling them and execute them.

Since I learned about healing the gut, avoiding foods I am allergic to, my mental status improved almost to what I was in Hong Kong when playing like a free monkey was everything. How true can it be that a good un-leaky gut can change my life. Now I am the one to remind my wife of little things at home. And I can remember things without using memory techniques to help very often.

Diet affecting the mental status is not just an observation by the physicians practicing Functional Medicine or diet professionals observing in their clients. The main point here is the wrong allergic foods causes inflammation in the whole body, as discussed in every chapter especially in chapter 42. Inflammation affecting the brain-functions has been the subjects of research studies, hundreds of them. Most studies showed improved mental status by avoiding high saturated fat, high fatty meats and starchy foods diet. Avoiding them, I regained my mental performance.

How did I know some foods are bad for me?

When I eat too much bread or eat too much sugar, I feel sleepy. And I feel an urge to defecate all the time as a reminder of the bowels being irritated and inflammed. When I drink milk or eat cheese, I have diarrhea. This milk intolerance is a result of allergy to these foods. It hurts the guts to the degree of diarrhea. So I avoided wheat products, milk and cheese, and sugar and salt as much as I can.

To enhance mood and memory, the most important foods are the green-leaf vegetables that I had a lot in Hong Kong. They have lots of fibers to bind away fats, toxins, sugars, hormones and carcinogens. One of these days, maybe I should think about periodic fasting too. That is part of life and "diet" of the Old Stone Age.

To sum up:

Diet that fills 80% of the stomach, of mainly vegetables without wheat, milk, sugar and meats had set up a low-inflammatory state in my whole adolescent body in Hong Kong.

The mental performance was excellent. But when I was an adult in America, the American diet of fast food, fat protein, milk and desserts have compromised my mental performance for almost 50 years. Though I have still been functioning well.

The worst of American diet is over-calorie which eventually is very inflammatory to the body. On the other end of the spectrum, feeling hungry like when I was an adolescent did wonders to my mental performance. Routine physical activities needed to burn the calorie, may help to cut down the harms of the American diet.

But finally, avoiding foods I am allergic to like milk, cheese, bread, and sugar, and tried hard to stop eating when I feel 80% full. I regained most of my clear mental performance.

Chapter Thirty Three - How I controlled my type-2 Diabetes and Weight, the healthy way.

I have type-2 diabetes, the adult-onset diabetes mellitus. So I am going to talk about my diabetic control as a patient, not as an expert like the endocrinologist who is my diabetic doctor. That is Dr Alice K. Lee, MD who is writing a real book on diabetics as a specialist in diabetic and hormonal diseases care. Alice and I worked in the same hospital 30 years ago.

How my diabetic was diagnosed and managed

It was in 1986 when my blood test showed a blood sugar test before breakfast was 146 mg/dL. Repeated test was 140 mg/dL, so diabetic was diagnosed. I was expecting the disease, because it runs in my family.

In the 1980's and early 1990's, the diabetic control was simple. After diagnosis, one can try diet and exercise control. If not successful, the oral medication (Metformin) would be used. If oral medication did not help to control sugar, I would need insulin injections.

Popular diabetes treatment in the 1980's

The popular treatment in clinical trials was "tight-control", using different types of insulin of various time-onset, and time-length-of- action in different combinations. The idea was to achieve very low normal glucose levels around the clock.

But not too soon this way of tight-glucose control was given up. A study showed patients with tight-control treatments had more mortality than the non-tight-control patients. Nobody wants a slightly higher chance of dying. Tight-control fell out of favor.

My diabetes was only fairly controlled, but I avoided insulin injections. Because I know my insulin level was already high. It is high in every type-2 diabetic patients. And high levels of insulin would be metabolically harmful and highly inflammatory (Insulin Growth Factor-1, IGF-1, that co-secreted out with insulin is very inflammatory). So I really did not want to make it higher. I had to make sure I exercise enough, avoid sugar and starchy foods, and eating till 80% full plus a cup of liquid to make me feel full. I thought that was enough to control the diabetes.

My diabetes was not controlled well. Weight was the problem

I was seeing an endocrinologist/internist in Canal Street, Manhattan. He was a physician who cared about patients very much. He found out for me I had sky-high HgA1c and flipped through my chart quickly and found the reason. I had gained 10 pounds since the last follow-up. Only then I learned what I should have known as a physician – not to gain weight as a diabetic patient. Because gaining weight is the worst thing in diabetic control, next to over-eating.

That forced me to start eating really 80% full, and maintain my exercise which was swimming every other day. My HgA1c since then had remained at low 7.0. That was not bad. It was fair control. Exercise is a good way to avoid diabetic nerve damage, kidney damage, and blood vessel damage. But obviously, I did not control the diabetes well at all because the HgA1c never was below 7.0. Below that level, diabetes is said to be in control. Once my HgA1c was higher than 8. What happened next is not a surprise when I went to see the eye doctor.

Does lost 10 pounds lead to better control of diabetes by itself? No.

After stopped eating as soon as I felt 80% full, and I had increased my lap-swimming, and continued with the mainly "lots of non-starchy vegetables" diet. I lost weight gradually. Eventually, I lost that 10 extra lbs and the HgA1C came down to 7.3.

But is it the weight loss alone that lowered my blood glucose level? Recent studies of inflammation showed it was the lowering inflammation that led to better diabetic control. Losing weight is associated with lowering internal inflammation.

What evidence supports lowering inflammation controls DM better?

Yes, two small studies showed there is a correlation of HgA1C to inflammation. One study of about 80 patients showed the lower the inflammation, the lower the HgA1c. Another study published in an American Diabetic Association (ADA) journal Diabetic Care in 2013 showed that as inflammation was lowered by active management of more than 400 patients, the HgA1c went down, and it is associated with significant fall in inflammation tests hsCRP (High sensitivity C-reactive protein).

DM patients do have a higher hsCRP in past studies. 42% in one study showed patients of DM-2 had hsCRP of more than 3 mg/L, in high risk for cardiovascular events.

A powerful weapon indeed to drastically lower blood sugar, by lowering internal inflammations, by, you guess what? By eating foods with good fats - (Olive, olive oil, avocados, nuts and seeds, dark chocolates, coconuts and coconut drinks in cartons from stores)

But eating good fats can lead to lowering of HgA1C too. This I discovered after reading a book by Mark Hyman, MD (30). Dr Hyman is highly respected in the world of Functional Medicine for his excellent scientific interpretations of the studies and principles of evidence-based functional medicine. Dr Hyman has more than 20,000 patients treated that way successfully, by eating good fats and lots of non-starchy veggies.

I am now starting to try that myself. I will list the good fats in chapter 39, titled Beneficial Statements (BS). One caution is, fat has twice the calorie per gram. So I would have to be careful not to eat too much good fats, no matter how good it is. Total calories still matters.

There was bleeding at the back of my eye (retina)

Shortly after my diabetes was poorly controlled, I went to have a routine eye doctor visit. It was discovered there was a bleeding couple of weeks before my visit to the eye doctor. The blood was still being absorbed. If it happened just a few millimeters away, the bleeding could have blinded my left eye which has been my good eye. The right eye was Ok.

It woke me right up. I got to control my diabetes well. Otherwise many complications of diabetes which were as serious as the retinal bleeding could happen. From that point on, my diabetes has been better controlled.

So what are the important things I had done to control diabetes? Let me put that on hold for a second till I mentioned how I made sure there would not be retinal bleeding again.

Things I did to avoid retinal bleeding again

I did a lot of praying, hoping I wouldn't go blind. Then I knew next I had to control my sugar level. High glucose (sugar) in blood generates free radicals. Radicals can damage any organ in my body. The tinniest "tissues" that can get heavy damages are the tiniest arteries and veins in the eyes and kidneys. Diabetes patients frequently have problems with eyes and kidneys, that is why.

While I was looking healthy and feeling healthy with high sugar in blood, diabetes was poorly controlled, I had the retinal bleeding since the tiny vessels got easily damaged. I absolutely avoided sweet sugary foods, avoided starchy foods that can turn right into sugar. This being potatoes I had to avoid. And eating till 80% full helped. More about this will be discussed later. I did not know about the importance of lowering the inflammation to control diabetes yet. This came later. I started taking herbal medications that were studied to strengthen the blood vessels. All those herbs that helped were all anti-inflammatory as well, as I later learned.

The herbs I took to control retinal hemorrhage (bleeding)

1. *Panax ginseng* – It healed blood vessel injuries in studies of hypertension damaging blood vessels. It might have teratogenic (baby malforming) effect. Pregnant women may have to avoid it. I avoid taking it after noon time. It may cause insomnia if taken late in the day.

2. *Bilberry* – In studies it prevented fragile vessels being formed. So only strong small arteries and veins would form. *Bilberry* has the nasty side effects of intoxication if taken on long term. I take it intermittently.

3. *Ginkgo biloba* – It increases blood flow by generating nitric oxide. Nitric oxide dilates blood vessels so they won't constrict to be in a position of more likely damaged by the increase current of blood flow. *Ginkgo's* anti-oxidant effect would lower inflammation.

Inflammation radicals can damage tiny blood vessels easily. *Ginkgo biloba* has ginkgoside that is poisonous if accumulated to a high level. I take it at regular dose indicated on the bottle, and never overdose myself on this one, so the drug has no chance of accumulating too high. High level of ginkgoside is known to be fatal.

4. Lutein and Zeaxanthine – Both are anti-oxidants. Both are carotenoids, belonging to vitamin A family. Their levels are very high in the retina. They are supposed to counter-act the UV light damage to the eyes. Both of these "vitamins" have been studied in two major NIH sponsored studies and proven effective to protect the eyes. They could stop the progression of macular degeneration, and cataract or reverse them. Both as vitamins can be found in a single supplement containing both vitamins, available on-line or in health food stores.

First and foremost for me is the weight control, the healthy way

As mentioned earlier in this chapter, I gained 10 pounds once and my diabetes was "out of control". My retinal bleeding most probably was due to poor control of diabetes at that period in my life. So I tried to eat 80% full all the time. But it is hard to do if I continued the habit of "cleaning the plate". The best thing was to walk away from the table when enough was eaten. But doing that was almost impossible without some tricks. I just drink soup or water when I'm 80% full, so right away it would become 100% full. My weight has been stable since.

I kept my weight on the lean-side of "standard weight"

My weight was 164 lbs when I was working. That was standard weight by formula. But for diabetes, perhaps a few pounds less is better. Then after the retinal bleeding, the weight eventually went down to 158 lbs. And there it remained till today.

What happened when I am 80% full? Weight-control to continue

Normally when we feel full after a meal without the addition of a cup of liquid distending the stomach, it is over-eating. When the stomach is really full, it will not tell the brain "I'm full". So we don't feel full and continue eating. The signal from the stomach of feeling full to reach the brain is delayed by 20 minutes later. In 20 minutes, people like my grandsons, could finish half a chicken. That's way over-eating, I always remind them the above piece of information. But they enjoyed their foods without blinking an eye at first, but later on after a few reminders, they at times ate 80% full. Teaching the young ones is our duty too.

The 20 minutes-delay might have its survival advantage through millions of years of evolution. It stored extra energy for the cave-men's emergency like running away from predators etc. If there were no emergency, they burned that extra-energy with their physical life-style of the old days anyway. But we modern humans never have a chance to burn the extra food we eat. We conveniently stored that extra-energy as fat on our belly. Yes, our liver diligently turned the extra-calories as fat for storage, preferentially at the belly. The foods that got turned into fat by the liver are excess carbohydrates, never fatty food themselves. So to cut down belly fat is to cut down excess carbohydrates, especially refined-carbs of flour, rice, and starchy foods.

So just drink that cup of liquid when I am 80% full. Would that work? Yes, it would work, even though I would feel hungry between meals. Hey! That's fasting. Feeling hungry is fasting and fasting is good, I'll explain later. But first, what did I do when feeling hungry?

What did I eat when feeling hungry between meals is the most important. (Some examples of good foods):

I ate things that switched the gene-on to burn fat. Yes, it has been studied. I just ate six walnuts with another cup of water. Walnuts are good fats with higher omega-3 (good fats) to omega-6 (bad Fats) ratio. It makes me feel full for a long time. Just like that, the walnuts started burning fat and in time, I'll be slim. Huh, how come?!

Walnuts have lots of omega-3 fats (like in fish oils). Omega-3 fats turned on our genes for fat burning, the researchers said. In fact, all good fats, good proteins will start fat burning also. Examples of some good fats are like fish oil, olives, olive oil, seeds and nuts, avocados, dark chocolates, and coconut meats and coconut oils. Good proteins are like fish, turkey, lean beef that are "grass-fed", eggs, nuts, seeds and sea foods. They have good fats and good proteins that burn our body-fats. Nuts are good for its fibers, and proteins, minerals and vitamins besides good fats. Nuts, like non-starchy vegetables, has high fiber content. Good bacteria in our gut extract energy from fibers and turned them into short chain fatty acids, stuff that help mend our leaky guts.

So fiber is of utmost importance. Commercial supplement-fiber is low in fiber contents weight to weight compared to foods. Fruits have twice the fiber than supplemental fiber, Non-starchy vegetables has eight times the fibers. Half or more of my plate at dinner is those vegetables.

Are all nuts the same?

All nuts are good for their fibers, minerals, fats and proteins. But some nuts have better ratios of good fat to bad fats. Omega-3 is good fat; omega-6 is not, it starts inflammation. Nuts high in omega-3 are walnuts, macadamia nuts, and pecans. The rest of the nuts have very high omega-6 content. But the rest of the nuts are good too, by comparison to other foods. Omega-6 taken with foods of high fiber content is less harmful.

If I have allergy to nuts, a lot of other foods can give me good fats or proteins that would start fat-burning, yes the fat on my belly to be burned. A salad with virgin olive oil, lumps of cooked chicken meats, a drink of fermented goat milk (read label), a small cup of coconut drinks, half of an avocado, and a cup of vegetable/fruit smoothie in the past (not now as it gives me diarrhea), or any good-fats, good-proteins snacks I can find in dietary books, an easy one are eggs. Eggs don't raise the bad small dense LDL. Eggs do raise the harmless large-size fluffy LDL. But the larger LDL is harmless. It is the small dense LDL that can dig under the inside surface of the vessel and starts plaque formation.

With this nifty way of snacking when I could not tolerate the hunger between meals, I successfully maintain my weight 6 lbs below my standard weight. And I did not become under-nutrition.

Fasting is eating about 50% of the regular amount of food. Do it one or two days per week per one of Dr Michael Mosley's book (9), will keep one trim and smart. I feel sorry I probably could never do that. But what good is it anyway? Are there lots of good things to come when one goes on fasting?

Benefit of intermittent fasting (Rather deeply scientific and speculative, skip if you want to. But it has its results)

Dr Mosley kept himself slim and smart with one day a week 50% calories fasting. What is the reason this worked? It probably has an ancient explanation. The Old Stone Age people had to hunt and pick fruits or vegetables when they started feeling hungry. They kept their hunger till the foods were found. That had been the way life for millions of years. Intermittent hunger was part of old-life for millions of years. In those days with repeated hunger periods, some set of gut bacteria evolved to "eat" mucus in the gut, the only food stuff that's available. Akkermansia bacteria species manage the mucus for energy. So the bacterial pattern was Akkermansia species dominant over the rest of the hundreds of species of bacteria (That together weights 3 to 5 lbs) during fasting. After a one person (Dr Mosley himself) fasting study, Dr Mosley showed Akkermansia dominance in the stool analysis.

So was the same finding shown by the American Gut Project (a study). Akkermansia is associated with leanness.

Weight-control means a lot of work as you can see from above.

It involves the discipline of calorie restriction (80% full diet), frequent exercises, having adequate sleep so the body can do its repair and maintenance; avoiding stresses with exercise, meditation when needed. And at last, as a retired physician, having no sleep-deprivations every four nights (on-call), it greatly helped. Sleep-deprivation is the main reason in America that brings stresses, studies showed.

Sleep deprivation also can fatten people up. I felt hungry after on-call with sleep deprivation, and ate a lot after. That was what studies show exactly. That sleep deprivation makes one hungry. Hungry off-meal time eating is the main reason for extra calories stored as fat. That was why I was 10 lbs heavier before retirement. That is why now I turned off the TV and sleep before 11 PM so I won't be sleeping too late and hurt myself with sleep deprivation. All these took four pounds off my pre-retirement weight of 164 pounds. But the achievement of more weight loss was made possible with anti-inflammatory treatments and calorie restriction by eating 80% full plus liquids to make it 100% full.

Various anti-inflammatory treatments:

Lowering inflammation is to lower insulin resistance so I can be more sensitive to insulin and use glucose more efficiently. The use of Metformin and Actos aims at increasing insulin sensitivity. Life-styles and herbs can achieve the same goals:

•**Exercise** – Exercise is the greatest method to lower inflammation to increase insulin sensitivity. Studies showed it lowered the inflammatory markers (the blood tests for inflammations) TNF-alpha and IL-6 (TNF-tumor necrosis factor; IL-6 – Interleukin-6).

•**Adequate sleep** – A university study showed sleep-deprivation is the number 1 reason Americans are stressed. Stress brings inflammation. I do meditation to relieve my stress. Exercise helped too.

Sleep deprivation depress our immune system badly. It is dangerous for health especially in months when flu/cold happens.

•**Calorie restriction (CR)** – And avoiding sugar, so the blood sugar (glucose) level won't be too high. High sugar generates free radicals for inflammation. In studies, CR was found to be anti-inflammatory.

•**Anti-inflammatory foods** – All good foods like those mentioned earlier are anti- inflammatory. I drank water with turmeric powder added. In one study, turmeric-cooked foods prevented diabetes in people who are pre-diabetic. Alas, that is too late for me, hopefully not for you.

•**Healing leaky guts to lower gigantic inflammation -**

We have already discussed a lot about this topic, especially in chapter one. But it is easy to summarize how I did not lose more pounds but my HgA1c went below 7.0. just by healing the leaky gut. First avoid bad foods, as described briefly in this chapter earlier. This healed my irritable bowel syndrome. My guts became tight and not leaky.

Since half of the colonic stool content is dead gut bacterial particles as analyzed in studies. When my guts were leaky, billions of bacterial particles got in my system. My immune system sent out cells to chase each particle, secreting inflammatory chemicals to burn them dead. This happened internally all over the body. Those chemicals made me very inflammatory inside. Internal inflammation made me very insulin resistant. That worsened my diabetes control. My HgA1c was always higher than 7.0.

But it was different when I avoided eating inflammatory foods. I ate goods foods as described earlier in this chapter and chapter 39. My gut healed itself and shut out all the bacterial particles. The immune system now does not have to fight anymore. The inflammatory chemicals secreted in large amount before now came down. Inflammation calmed down.

My HgA1c went down as inflammation went down

The key event was, as my internal inflammation went down. The insulin resistance went down. So was my HgA1c. It went down below 7.0 for the first time in two decades. At this level, the American Diabetic Association said the sugar is controlled.

As my immune system does not put out too much burning chemicals anymore, all my organs became more normal and function more effectively. My blood sugar went down as they were more effectively utilized by different organs. Lower sugar level internally means the liver would not convert as much of the extra glucose to fat. My fat in the belly went down a little. I did not lose additional weight because I am already 6 pounds below standard weight.

After my HgA1c went below 7.0, I thought eating good fats was really the key for my diabetic control. So to make it better, I increased eating nuts, and coconut drinks to try to get my HgA1c even lower. But I forgot about total calorie increase by this behavior. A surprise was in waiting.

Back to the basics of diabetes control, no sugar, no over-calories. Because controlling internal inflammation alone is not going to cut it.

Since lowering my internal inflammation brought my HgA1c below 7, in a range of "controlled" per American Diabetes Association. I thought lowering inflammation was all I need to control my diabetes further and I slacked off my 80% full when eating. I ate more "good fats" and good proteins. These foods are calorie dense

Right before my next check up of diabetes, it made me feel glad because I expected another lower HgA1c number. But it turned out to be 7.5. That was a disappointment. I didn't know what happened. I continued avoiding bad foods. Signs were showing my internal inflammation was under good control: My skin looked good, no acne ever appeared, no diarrhea and feeling good-mood all the time. So my inflammation has been well-controlled. Theoretically my HgA1c should keep on going down. But that was not the case. Instead, the HgA1c went up.

So in addition to controlling inflammation, I have to keep other diabetes-control maneuvers. Going through the laboratory results, my diabetic doctor, Dr Lee showed my good cholesterol (HDL) went down too. That was most probably the result of my slacking off on the routine exercises which is known to increase HDL, the good cholesterol. It made me realize my tight exercise schedule was necessary for my diabetes control too. And my eating more good fats was a problem also. Even good fats carry a lot of calories. So for the future, I will have to exercise more, eat a bit less of the good fats and good proteins.

So calorie restriction (Eating 80% full) plus non-starchy vegetable being the dominant amount of food is really an important principle of diabetes control. I will strive to make my HgA1c below 7.0.

To sum up:

The most important thing in controlling my diabetes, in the classical way, was my weight control. Weight control involved calorie restriction by eating 80% full, exercise, adequate sleep, and avoiding stress. Doing the above kept my weight down to 158 lbs. So weight control and calorie control remain the most important steps in diabetic control.

Chapter Thirty Four - A few words on Alzheimer's Disease

A physician's father is developing Alzheimer's Disease

An old friend who is a practicing physician asked me about best treatment for Alzheimer's Disease (AD). Her friend, another physician, was wondering what useful treatment there was for AD. His father was developing AD. They were not sure the current conventional treatment for controlling symptoms of AD was what they wanted. The current treatments do control AD symptoms. And the qualities of life for the patients are better. But such treatments do not delay the progression of AD. No conventional medication is capable of delaying the progression of AD.

These physician friends knew I have been studying supplements for a while and they knew available treatments are only for symptoms control. So they were eagerly looking for alternatives.

I am not an expert at all in treating AD. But I remembered two large studies using high dose Vitamin E has delayed the progression of AD by 6, and 7 months respectively The study that delayed the disease for 6 months were gold standard study involving 600 VA hospital patients in Minnesota. And the quality of life was even better than available treatments. At 2000 International Units (IU) of vitamin E (alpha-tocopherol) daily, there were no serious side effects, even though potentially such high dose could increase risk of bleeding and increase cholesterol levels. And if taken on long term for many years, could increase prostate cancer risk and intracranial bleeding. This particular VA study only had an average follow up of 2.3 years.

In this case, I was involved in just a conversation, so I did not have follow-up news on the "father".

Diet-based anti-inflammatory treatment studies for AD:

With diet based anti-inflammatory treatments being more and more popular, more and more small-scale studies were done and proved positive in improving chronic diseases including AD, the National Institute of Health (NIH) of the United States is conducting large scale interventional trials to see if Mediterranean-like diets can benefit Alzheimer's Disease. These trials are actively enrolling patients. The future of diet-based treatments seems getting more and more relevant. There is no surprise that these kinds of treatments may work well to stop the progression or even to prevent AD. AD is one big inflammatory disease. Persistently in the blood and spinal fluids of AD patients, inflammation can be detected: The inflammatory marker test TNF-alpha had been found to be always elevated. Enrolling in such studies is a real good way to be treated, hoping for big delay of progression or prevention by Mediterranean diets. Therefore diet may help control AD, but is being studied only.

Hypothetically, there may be another very effective treatment for AD, but needs even small studies to be done to prove whether it has any merit:
In about 90% of AD patients' blood and spinal fluid, persistently there is the presence of spirochetes. The bacteria can cause an infection resulting in a chronic inflammation. There are two chronic diseases like that by spirochetes. We know one spirochete can cause tertiary syphilis affecting the brain and cognitive functions chronically. It could lead to mental deterioration like AD. Another spirochete cause Lyme's Disease chronically affecting the central nervous system too. Both could be fatal at the end, like AD. The same or another spirochetal bacteria can easily infect people and chronically cause AD too. It's hard to imagine it is just so easy, but a course of antibiotics may tell and may just offer a cure for AD. Though this sounds rather like a dream. But only large scale studies will tell whether it is just a dream or whether it is dream comes true. Isn't it?
There are available antibiotics for spirochetes by now from experiences of treating Borrelia burgdorferi that caused the Lyme's disease at its disseminated stage. A clinical trial may save millions of lives and save billions of dollars for AD care. Anybody wants to be the savior?

To sum up:
AD is an inflammatory disease now the NIH of the United States is enrolling patients for diet-based trials. Two large studies with vitamin E were able to delay the onset for 6, and 7 months.

Chapter Thirty Five – How I controlled my Carpel Tunnel Syndrome

How I got my Carpel Tunnel Syndrome (CTS):

I got it from using the computer typing for lectures, for patients' medical histories, and for writing books all my life. I did not learn the ergonomics of typing and my hands were lower than the computer keyboard. Fortunately, I only got a mild case of mainly pain on my wrists, the right wrist hurt worse than the left. Though my right hand fell asleep a few times when I was sleeping, but that probably does not mean I injured my median nerve seriously to the degree my hands fell sleep totally. I woke up and my hand woke right up. That was not bad because it only hurts rarely.

If your CTS is a lot worse, have it taken care by a professional. The best thing for severe CTS is to have surgery which has a successful rate of 90%. Otherwise losing the median nerve and the efficient function of the hands is a very pitiful thing. Of course, that refers to disabling CTS which I don't have.

What treatment I used?

The conventional non-surgical treatment is non-steroidal anti-inflammatory drugs (NSAID) and water pills (diuretics). I never use them because my case is mild compared to the risk of the side effects of the above two drugs. NSAID can cause stomach ulcers. It gave me sharp pain in the stomach as soon as I took one in years past. The diuretics dehydrate, not good for my internal organs, especially the kidneys. With diabetes, chronic dehydration could cause renal failure.

But one antioxidant supplement I used might have made the disease a lot milder. It was alpha lipoic acid (ALA). It is a master anti-oxidant our body makes to neutralized radicals and inflammations. I called it a master anti-oxidant because it can rejuvenate all the other antioxidants in the body. Taken as a supplement, it was effective in relieving the neuropathy (nerve disease) of diabetes in studies. So I used it for a year to help neutralizing radicals in my body. I had no neuropathy. But it ended up causing me a lot. My gray hair was turning white (see chapter 18), so I stopped it. But it seemed that since then, my CTS almost never gave me real pain in the wrists again, till I was typing a lot while writing this book. So maybe ALA did heal my CTS a lot? But at what price? That I would never know as no one knows about the harms of ALA overdose for a year could do.

But now the computer is about an inch below my elbow. It does not add to the old injury on my carpel tunnel. Yet the repeated typing did worsen the old injury in the carpel tunnel on the right hand. I was feeling a mild pain in my sleep. But one thing I did prevented the pain at night.

Keeping the wrist warm at night prevented the mild CTS pain in my right wrist

One thing I did succeeded in preventing the pain in my right wrist at night or whenever I feel the pain of the wrist. I wore a pain of cotton fingerless gloves that covered the wrist, thus keeping them warm at night or in the day when necessary. It is like arthritis pain that disappears in the summer when the weather is warm. Gloves keep my wrists warm and keep the pain away.

Is it ALA or anti-inflammatory diet I am adopting eased the pain?

This question will never be answered because the pain has been rare and mild. It is hard to quantify. But if the NSAID worked by reducing the body's inflammation, it is reasonable to assume lowering the internal inflammation with the "good foods" would help decrease the pain frequency in my wrists. Lowering internal inflammation has been found to lower symptoms of arthritis in thousands of patients, including myself.

The anti-inflammatory foods are: Good fats, good proteins, and good carbohydrates. Examples of some good fats are like fish oil, olives, olive oil, seeds and nuts, avocados, dark chocolates, and coconut meats and coconut oils. Good proteins are like fish and sea foods, turkey, lean beef that is "grass-fed", eggs, and nuts and seeds. They have good fats and good proteins that burn our body-fats. Nuts are good for its fibers, good fats and proteins, minerals and vitamins. Nuts, like non-starchy vegetables, has high fiber content. Good bacteria in our gut extract energy from fibers and turned them into short chain fatty acids, stuff that help mend our leaky guts. No leaky guts, no inflammations. (See chapter 1, 9 &42)

So fiber is of utmost importance. Supplement fiber is low in fiber weight to weight compared to foods. Fruits have twice the fiber than supplement fiber. Non-starchy vegetables have eight times the fibers. Half my plate at dinner is those vegetables. Of course, one has to avoid the bad foods to begin with. (See chapter 39)

To sum up:

For severe, disabling Carpel Tunnel Syndrome, I advise to talk to a hand-surgeon. For mild CTS like mine, I just wear a pair of fingerless gloves to keep my wrist warm when I am sleeping, that is when the pain comes because the night is colder. The gloves keep my hands warm. This simple maneuver works for me.

Avoiding bad foods, eating good foods to lower internal inflammation is important lifestyle that helped control arthritis pain, which CTS is one.

Chapter Thirty Six - How I prevent Cramps and Pain in my Calf of the lower Legs.

These leg clamps are called "charley horses". Mine may be due to a little bad circulation, or more likely, and more often, due to over-exercises.

When I swam too much, the leg cramps happened often, I would just stop swimming and stretched my legs a few seconds. Then all was good. Sometimes, I could even swim a little more after the exercise-related cramps were over. One time, when I did that, I almost choked with water. It is advisable to just finish with swimming when cramps happen.

Hundreds of cramps due to (over) swimming were easily taken care:

After 50 to 70 laps swimming in the pool, I often came down with cramps in the calf, in the past, when I did not do flutter kicks correctly, usually in the right calf. Those leg cramps were easily taken care of. I just swam to the end of the pool, grabbed the edge of the pool, and put my toes against the wall, and stretched my legs by lifting my body away and slightly up from the wall. The stretching always got rid of the cramps right away. What is the mechanism of cramps? There are many speculations you won't be interested to know. But when too much exercise is done, the relaxing phase is prolonged. If I push hard before the muscles finishes relaxation, cramps can happen. Whatever it is, I can relax and leave the pool after the cramps were over, or sometimes, took a risk of drowning and continued swimming. Of course, in the pool for a good swimmer, the risk of drowning is very low. And there are the life-guards, sitting high up watching over everybody.

So each time before the cramp fully went through its whole course, I terminated it by stretching. I never fully realized how awfully painful a charley horse cramp can be till one time I let it run its course.

When the muscle cramp went through the whole course,

the pain is excruciating:

For hundred of leg cramps I had before due to a little over swimming, I stretched the legs, and made them go away at once. So I thought cramps are something not to be afraid of. Till this one time, I was gathering data for this book with full concentration (an hour after I swam 70 laps, including using flippers). A muscle cramp threatened to happen at the dorsal surface (top surface) of my right foot. I thought it could be easy to take care of later. So I ignored it and continued editing. Half an hour later, I found out how horrible a completed muscle cramp could be. The whole right foot seemed to be on fire, any movement would hurt like hell. I was totally physically disabled. This happened right before bedtime after I drank a lot of water too after exercise. I lay in bed with the foot uncomfortably resting on a soft pillow. The posture was comfortable, but not the hell-fire-like pain. It continued without any sign of stopping. I had to take a Codeine pill for the pain which was the first time in three decades.

Needless to say, I could not fall asleep for three hours due to the pain. Finally, the heat generated by the warm blanket, and the effect of the Codeine together finally put me to sleep.

And needless to say, the lesson learned is "To terminate the cramp by stretching" as soon as the cramping starts by stretching the muscles fibers and prevent them from contracting abnormally to cause great pain.

Don't ever let the cramp run its full course.

But if this fails, and the cramping is serious, going to the emergency room to be evaluated by a professional is the advice of a reasonable next step. There are a few medications that can relax the muscles.

Early morning cramps are something else, the cold agglutinins

In the past, often during a peaceful sleep, these charley horses came galloping in, and the sharp pain woke me right up. Fortunately, I found a way to rein in those horses, and avoided being waken up every night. Yes, in the past, I had those painful cramps every night, usually early in the morning when I was sleeping. The early morning hours before waking up are usually the coldest time of the day in Long Island, New York. One possible cause for those early morning cramps might be due to a rarely known reason, the cold agglutinins.

I think my "cold-agglutinins" had been causing all those "charley horses" in the morning hours: Keeping the body-parts warm is the key

Normal leg cramps can be due to poor circulation, a pinched nerve in the spine, dehydration, over-use, lacking sufficient electrolytes like calcium, magnesium, or potassium. So if you have frequent leg cramps like me. It is time you go to see a doctor. But by eliminating all the above causes, I still had early morning leg cramps.

Then I was forced to consider something I leaned in the specialty of blood diseases called hematology. This I leaned from hematology textbooks. There is some protein that everybody has in their circulation. Some people have more, others have less of those proteins. These proteins are sub-units of antibodies that the immune system uses to fight infections.

These protein sub-units are a little abnormal. When they circulate to a colder part of the body like the legs, they stick to each other into clumps. They are called "cold agglutinins". These protein-clumps slow down circulation, cutting down the supply of oxygen and nutrients. If the fingers were affected, they turned blue and pale, and give out pain. This is called cold-agglutinins disease (with Raynaud's Phenomenon). It is a disease most doctors are not totally familiar in details. Can the clumps in my legs in the cold night hours gave me the clamps?

I believe my leg cramps were due to the cold agglutinins. Because I know I have a lot of those agglutinins which is associated with a few diseases. Hepatitis is one of the diseases that are associated with cold agglutinins. I am a carrier of hepatitis B acquired when I was being born. I acquired the hepatitis while passing through my mom's birth canal. She was a hepatitis B carrier too. Carrier state of hepatitis B used to be very common, as high as 80% in some population in the south of China in the old days.

Keeping my calves warm with old socks (without the toes part of the socks) took care of those early morning cramps

Those cold agglutinins gave me big charley horses in the calves every night. That is, until I cut the toe parts of my old socks and started wearing those hollow socks without ends during sleep, nicely wrapping around my calves. This kept my lower legs warm and there was no more leg cramps waking me up at night anymore. I usually also cover my lower legs with very thin blankets to make sure it would not be too warm to my legs, ended up the blanket being kicked off during sleep.

This self-treatment of the cold agglutinins induced ischemia (reduced blood flow) and pain was done in my forties. So it is definitely not ischemia due to poor circulations. When I was forty-something, it was too young for poor circulation related ischemia.

Everybody has certain amount of those cold-agglutinins, the book says. So it may help you to try a loose sock without ends to warm your lower legs during your sleep if you have charley horses there. It may just help you avoid leg cramps.

To sum up:

For exercise related cramps, I easily stretched my legs and made them go away. So terminating a cramp before it gets set is the best treatment. But one time I let the cramp run its course and later the pain almost killed me. It made me crawl on all fours going to the bathroom, avoiding the use of the feet with "hell-fire" pain. (I never realized it was just so easy to crawl like a baby again).

For otherwise regular morning cramps in the legs, that I thought are due to cold-agglutinins, I wear a pair of loose sock without the toe ends (by cutting the toe-parts away). Wear it on the calves of the legs during sleep. It may get rid of the nightly leg cramps. But please be mindful that too frequent a leg cramps may mean a serious underlying diseases that needs a doctor's attention as soon as possible.

Chapter Thirty Seven – *Aloe* healed Decubitus Ulcers and stop Hemorrhoidal Pain

Non-healing decubitus ulcers healed by *Aloe vera*

Once I discussed with a professional friend about drugs on wound-healing. He mentioned even large wounds with denuded skins now can use artificial skin to cover a large wound area. This was impossible in the past for large skin wounds.

I mentioned to him *Aloe vera* can heal those wounds too if the *Aloe vera* juice is spread on the new dressing change. It would kill even broad-spectrum antibiotic-resistant bacteria and healed the wound. I mentioned that casually because I saw an *Aloe vera* plant growing in his porch. I commented that the *Aloe vera* besides antibacterial, is also antiviral, and anti-fungal. And it heals tissues also.

A few months later, the friend told me over the phone excitedly that the *Aloe vera* "saved his life". He has hemorrhoids. For two days, he could hardly walk because of the sharp pain. He tried every pain medication he had at home. It only helped very little. The pain was due to the infected hemorrhoids. I reminded him of *Aloe vera* not too long ago for hemorrhoid pain. So in order to kill the bacteria that infected the hemorrhoids and caused the excruciating pain, he cut a piece of *Aloe vera* in the form of a small stick, removed most of the skin, leaving a strip of linear skin for support of the jelly-like *Aloe vera* inside, and inserted it into the inside of the anus gently, avoiding bursting the hemorrhoids. Right away, the hemorrhoidal sharp pain was gone. He was able to walk without pain.

Another case of sharp pain relief

To make the story short, there was another case of hemorroidal pain inactivated another brave wife to be bed-bound and suffering. The same way of cure was achieved in another friend's wife.

Two cases convinced me that *Aloe vera's* antibiotic effect could really save people from severe pain due to infection of the skin. I am thinking whether antibiotic ointment that is readily available in drug stores could probably do the same. But to find a vehicle of carrying the antibiotic ointment for anal pain is impossible, and I also wonder would the antibiotic ointment be strong enough to do the job.

Chapter Thirty Eight – My Cautions in taking Herbs

Herbs have always been powerful to me

I was born in a poor village in southern china, I was always ill as a child. Herbs came to my rescue each and every time. In fact, it was the herbs that helped me survived a dozen of very serious illness with cold shaking chills and fever, headache and a huge amount of crying. In all fairness, if not for the herbs, I won't be here writing this book. As a physician now, I would recognize these as critical illnesses. There were no Intensive Care Units where I was, in the poor rural country-side of southern China.

My mom became a healer in my critical illnesses like that. Unceremoniously, my mom would rub on a good amount of "Tiger Balm" ointment on my forehead, the temporal areas, and the whole neck, ignoring my crying and protesting because of the pungent smell and the burning of the balm. Then she covered me with three thick blankets. Then there came the most important step, she would insist on me not to get out of the blankets. Otherwise I would face death-penalty – dying from the illness. Anyway, she sat by the bedside there to watch till I fell asleep. That was all it took to cure me. I figured out this cure was less than 50 cents.

Just what happened? Wait a minute, isn't that child-abuse? Slapping some smelly ointment on a sick child, cover him with three thick blankets, then leave him alone? Even the busiest of us medical men wouldn't dare do that. Those were the old days, my friend.

Hilariousness aside, scientifically, what did I think happen? The "Tiger Balm" contains a lot of herbal constituents. One of them is clove oil which is also a Western herb that is antibacterial, antiviral, and antifungal. After the three blankets covered my body and head totally, the warmth made me feel more comfortable, the chill went away. The body heat with fever evaporated the clove oil-containing herb-ointment called the "Tiger Balm", I breathed in the vaporized herbs which started killing the viruses or bacteria that caused the illness in my respiratory tract. Under the three blankets, elevated temperature developed with the high fever, High temperature denatured (broke up) protein coats of the viruses and they died. So heat was perhaps the main force that killed the virus. (That was why I never ordered Tylenol for patients with fevers unless they felt very uncomfortable with the fever). When I woke up, I would feel normal with no fever and the illness would be gone. It was time for me to play again. So I always believe in the power of the herbs.

My mom and the elders always pointed out deadly herbs to me

One of the herbs happened to be a delicious food too. It was the *Ginkgo biloba* nuts. Each autumn, thousands of *Ginkgo* nuts fell from the tree onto the ground. Eventually the seeds were there for the picking. Mom used it for cooking. It tasted so good when cooked with soybean thin-bread (soft), seasoned by soybean paste. I always continued to eat them up without stop. That's the time my mom would sternly stop me from eating more than six or seven seeds. I thought that was child abuse at the time. But now I understood, when consuming more than ten seeds, one could vomit due to nausea, could have seizures, or rarely, one could die. Now I understand that wasn't child abuse. My mom knew the *Ginkgo* seeds could be poisonous if consumed too much due to the toxin Ginkgoside.

Another lesson I learned happened when I was near my retiring age. In the campus of the University of California at Davis, I took seven inch-long tips of the *California Ephedra* that stopped my "tearful-crying" due to hay fever. The "crying" stopped. But due to the herb, I had a short run of irregular heart-beats. This could be the fatal irregular heart-beats that *Ephedra* can do. That is why it is banned by most countries in the world, because dangerous herbs are potentially fatal.

What the herbal gurus advised when taking herbal drugs:

As I said before, always run it by professional who is knowledgeable with herbal medicines. So he/she can evaluate your liver status to see if the liver can metabolized the herb, see if your kidneys can excrete the herb, see if you would have drug-interactions with the herb, and if you are allergic to the drug.

If you have asthma or hay fever, you may be prone to allergies. Herbal drugs can be very allergenic. A harmless herb that is thought to be safe except in people who are allergic to grass or flowers, like *Echinacea*, after being used by millions of people. Some serious allergic type of reaction has been reported to cause liver failure and kidney failure, in two case-reports. Thus if you start taking a new herb after a professional consultation, but if you feel sick, stop the herb and see a professional. Or if you start to feel breathing difficulty or serious dizziness after taking herbs in a short period of time, call an ambulance to rush you to the Emergency Room. Other similar serious and sometime dangerous signs include swelling of the lips and the mouth and throat, with or without big generalized rash all over the body. That is the time to call an ambulance if serious.

Here are more important points from me and the herbal gurus. They are not all inclusive.

1. Be aware they are medications. They have side effects and drug interactions.
2. No herbs to take during breast feeding or pregnant.
3. Infants and the elderly don't handle herbs well. It is unsafe for them. (Biologically, I'm not elderly yet).
4. Stop herbs one to two weeks before surgery. Most of them increase bleeding risk. Some can make glucose adjustment impossible.
5. Check "PDR for Herbal Medicine" from libraries to see contra-indications, precautions and drug interactions.
6. Herbs could mess up anesthesia, increase bleeding, or make control of sugar in the blood difficult during anesthesia. So make sure to mention it to surgeons and the anesthesiologists before scheduling surgery. Herbs to be stopped 2 weeks before surgeries.
7. Take herbs or supplements only when you know you are deficient. Superfluous supplements have been shown to cause cancers. These were reports from major "golden" studies. Supplement like beta-carotenes has increased risk of lung cancer, high dose vitamin E long term had increased risk of prostate cancer, folate (folic acid) for colon cancer-recurrence prevention had increased colon cancer instead.
8. Herbs are for short term use only, maybe unsafe long term.
9. Begin taking herbs with low dose and stop at low dose if it works already. If it does not work at recommended dose, discontinue it.

Part Two

New Sciences

Chapter Thirty Nine - Beneficial Statements: Good and bad foods Good and bad Lifestyles.

BS in this chapter represents beneficial statements

BS is an abbreviation that everybody knows. Because it also is an abbreviation that stands for "bull-shit" - a negative impolite slang meaning "Saying things that are really indeed meaningless". But now BS here means "beneficial statements". So one of these days, you would say to yourself, let me see Dr J.'s "BS" of how to lower my internal inflammation to get rid of my pimples. Or you may suddenly think about my "BS" that said processed foods are bad. You may refrain from grabbing it in the store. So these "BS's is designed for you to easily recall there are some beneficial statements (BS) that even can help prevent cancers. And that's for real. So please enjoy reading the beneficial statements in this chapter repeatedly.

Thanks to the gurus' books. Otherwise these BS are available only to the ears of the privileged few who have lots of money.

The vibrant and healthy body

There is a trilogy of the ideal body – The physical body, the spirit and the activity. Each part is important. Two parts of our vibrant healthy body are affected by the foods we eat. Yes, besides the physical body, the spirit is affected by foods as well.

Good foods can give us good mood, without mood swings, without depression, and the head being clear without brain fog. These are not only proven scientifically, hundreds of thousands of patients can tell you it is so. I am a happy witness to that as you can see from the different chapters in this book. So if you eat those good foods, or more importantly, avoid those bad foods, you may obtain the same status of mind in as soon as two weeks. Give it a trial, you will be a believer. So it is important to learn just what foods are bad and what foods are good.

Simple Recipe for Success of losing weight and lowering HgA1C, if you are overweight

It is this simple: Fill the meal plates to more than half a plate of non-starchy cooked vegetables and fill the remaining of the plate with good fats and good proteins. And one most important thing for lowering HgA1c is eating 80% full and to drink some liquid, then you will feel full and not over-eat. Form this habit and you will lose some weight and lower your HgA1c.

The rest of the chapter is for good foods and bad foods. Though sometimes, good or bad foods to you may depend on your sensitivity to the foods.

Most gurus said exercise is a must. Though a few gurus said exercise is even optional. (To them, avoiding bad foods would be enough to achieve good health and weight control).

Good foods or bad foods? Past confusions have been cleared up

Thousands of food studies were done. More than 500 key good studies helped defined good foods and bad foods. Most nutrition gurus agree on most good and bad foods. Only foods like beans, grains, legumes, eggs, coconut oils, and nightshade family of vegetables are not well defined as good or bad. If not consumed in large quantities, and not being sensitive to them, they could be good too. Otherwise, the rest of the common foods we eat are clearly good or clearly bad. So I am able to list them into two different food groups later in this chapter.

Both eggs and coconut oil have been exonerated. They are Ok to eat or drink. They belong to good foods category.

Individual sensitivity to a food defined bad food for me too

But again, even one clearly defined bad food, wheat and wheat flour products that contain gluten responsible for leaky gut syndrome is not necessary bad. 20% of people can eat them without problem. I can eat quite a bit of bread at one sitting without having my leaky gut syndrome coming back (of course, I won't eat bread every day, may be couple of times per month). This is a matter of individual sensitivities to that particular food. So how can I tell what is bad food for me. It is very easy to tell. If after I eat some food, and soon I feel brain-fog coming right back to me or worse still, diarrhea comes right back. Then this particular food is bad for me. Greasy foods in the restaurant always bring diarrhea back to me. I had to order non-greasy foods in the restaurants. Here, the offending stuff for diarrhea from food causing irritable bowel syndrome is always the trans fats. Milk does the same for me. Yet a lot of people can tolerate milk without any problem. Milk intolerance is a very common problem among people from non-Northern European origin. 80% of people are sensitive to milk in African Americans and Asians.

Foods I personally avoided that led to the transformation of a better health

1. **Milk and cheese** – Ask people with serious autoimmune diseases that got cured with "functional Medicine" physicians, they will tell you it is poison to them. To me, milk and cheese guarantee an urgent bathroom run for diarrhea. I used the enzyme lactase, it did not help. It was not good for me, I do have an allergy to milk. Avoiding them is probably necessary anyway. I avoided them almost a 100%.

2. **Bread and wheat product** - Gluten in the bread made of wheat flour does not seem to cause me a "leaky gut syndrome" like in the patients with serious autoimmune diseases, provided I eat them only very occasionally. These breads I referred to are hot Italian or French bread served up in restaurants. I do opt for sour dough or whole wheat bread without added sugar if available. 80% of people are sensitive to gluten to various degrees. Though only 5% develops celiac disease.

3. **Sugar** – I avoid it 100%. You can see why as you read on in this chapter under the heading of "bad foods". I avoided them a 100%. Ripen fruits are full or sugar, and should be included in the avoidance as well as any food that is very sweet.

4. **Salt** – I never add salt in my food nor cook with salt. It is inflammatory. Inflammation is the root of all diseases including heart attack, strokes, and even cancer as well as mild daily diseases like asthma, arthritis and more.

5. **Saturated fats and trans fats** – It causes inflammation that brought heart attacks right away in a lot of famous people who died after meals. Immediately after consumption of saturated fat in a meal, or meals cooked with a lot of trans fats, the inflammation they brought activate the clotting system, it can clot up the already narrowed arteries of the heart and cause an

heart attack or stroke.

Food additives I avoid – These food additives are high fructose corn syrup (HFCS) and trans fats. Now let's define what they are:

HFCS(sweet!) – High fructose corn syrup is the sweetener in all processed foods. Fructose is bad. Unlike regular sugar that gives the liver a choice of spending the sugar as energy, or turning it into triglycerides, or storing it as fat. Fructose gives the liver no choice but to store it as fat. In fact, it can get stored in the liver itself, and HFCS is the main cause of the epidemic "fatty liver disease". Storing fat is the main cause of obesity in USA where studies found most Americans obtain a major part of the daily calories from HFCS.

Since it is known to be bad by a lot of people, a new HFCS is made and was just labeled as "Fructose".

Trans fats – It is just vegetable oils with hydrogen forced into its molecular structure. It is tasty as all fats are when mixed with other food ingredients. It is cheaper than oil, and it extends the shelf life of the processed foods. So it is no wonder the choice of fat for food manufacturers. It is found in all processed foods in the stores and all baked goods. Why should HFCS and trans fats be found in all processed foods? Why not? The purpose of making processed food is to hook you up so you eat them again and unable to stop eating sometimes. Processed foods are all made with high sugar, fat and salt. So that is why they are all tasty. All these tasty additives are highly inflammatory, and dangerous to health.

In food-conferences meetings, I read that, to "Hook you up" is the only goal. How to do that are the topics of the conferences. So I just stop eating processed foods 99%, I hate to be hooked up, like an ox being led through the market by a string through the nose. This has something to do in me to yearn "To be free" and to be healthy.

Some foods are bad for almost all people, especially if taken in large amount

These are food with gluten in wheat products, sugar, perhaps milk, salt and bad fats, trans-fats and the processed foods with high content of it, high fructose corn syrup (HFCS) or simply called fructose in almost all processed foods. So I stay away from these processed foods as much as I can. This chapter would describe what scientists have proven as bad foods, and good foods. Also, life styles can be good or bad too. Some will be mentioned.

Bad foods-and the reasons why they are bad, presented in random statements:

Cheese

This food just came to my mind first. It does not mean bad food number one. It is bad because it increases the risk of breast cancer.

On 10/9/19, twelve thousand physicians from "Physician Committee for Responsible Medicine" demonstrated in Washington DC to urge the FDA to require adding label to cheese as a risk factor for breast cancer. Because form the study called "Life after Cancer Epidemiological study, 49% increased in death risk was seen in women with breast cancer treated, and consumed cheese a lot. That made national headline news.

The scientific explanation is straightforward. All the toxins and hormones the cow eat or given, got concentrated in the milk fat. Cheese is made by again concentrating the cow milk protein and fat. And bad things dissolve in fats. As the cows are fed hormones especially estrogens, and growth hormones, antibiotics, and the toxins-contaminating cattle-feeds they eat, got concentrated in the process of making cheese. Studies generally found the level of estrogens to be a risk factor for breast cancers.

When eating cheese, eat a lot of vegetables that contain lots of fibers. That may bind some of the hormones and toxins away. But it is still important to cut down on eating vast amount of cheese.

Sweeteners

It increases insulin resistance which is associated with obesity. One study showed taking it for one week, the insulin resistance appeared. It also decreases the good bacteria Akkermansia, the gut bacteria associated with leanness. At the same time, it increases bad gut bacteria secreting inflammatory molecules.

Trans-fats – Modified vegetable oil enabled foods to stay on shells for a long time.

In studies, it slowed down metabolism (we get fat), decreases fat burning, and increases cholesterol. It increases chances of strokes and heart attacks by clogging up arteries. Trans fat is also in every processed food to make them taste good. Lots of sugar, fat and salt makes processed foods taste good. Sugar, trans fat, and salt are all inflammatory. Big food manufacturers are required to give up trans fat in the manufacturing process. But restaurants are in a sense exempted. I only order non-greasy foods in restaurants.

HFCS – High fructose corn syrup, or simply labeled as fructose. It is most dangerous because it is in every processed food, soda, salad dressing, canned fruit, bread etc. It is used because it is very sweet and cheap to use. It is bad because it turned right into fructose in our body, and the liver convert it to fat. It is the number one reason for "fatty liver diseases" which can be fatal,

Trans-fats – The hydrogenated vegetable oil appears again for another vice characteristics. It can turn on a molecular switch in our cells to make more than 100 inflammatory chemicals. Good foods can turn it off, like eating omega-3 would turn off the switch called NFkB. These chemicals increase inflammation in our body. Internal inflammation is the cause for all chronic diseases including the metabolic syndrome which is associated with consumption of trans fats.

One piece of dense white bread - can turn on NFkB. Yes, white bread is inflammatory.

Saturated fat – This villain food looks harmless but ugly. But once you eat it, there is immediate blood vessel dysfunction predisposing to heart attack. That's why a lot of heart attacks appeared after fatty meals. Not to say it is conveniently stored as fat in your belly, and give rise to "remnant particle" that builds up plaques in the arteries.

If the anti-inflammatory fats omega-3 is high in blood, and at the same time, saturated fats actually can be anti-inflammatory when consumed together. It is also anti-inflammatory if eaten with foods containing lots of fibers. But I never want to take that chance of a heart attack regardless of what the researchers found. I stay away from saturated fat as much as I can.

Bad carbohydrates – Those vegetables that have a lot of sugar or a lot of starch are bad vegetables (carbohydrates). They made people hungry and get fat. This fact was demonstrated in a Harvard Obesity Study. In fact, all fruits when ripen, are full of sugar and are bad carbohydrates. I only dare eating a small piece or none at all each time.

High glycemic index (GI) carbohydrates, the ones that taste very sweet generally, and can turn into sugar quickly in the body system, are bad besides raising blood sugar, they eventually raise all the bad cholesterols. All ripen fruits are high GI foods. Five servings a day is really too much sugar for anyone to take. Sugars are like poisons to me.

Refined carbohydrates like rice and wheat flour without the bran, fibers and nutrients are just sugar in disguise. Sugar is another refined carbohydrate. A lot of bad things can happen with sugar as we shall see soon.

Vegetable oils

In a few decades in the past, they were found to lower cholesterol. But one randomized study showed no difference in heart attack deaths. Now sciences found that the vegetable oils contained a lot of omega-6, which is inflammatory, conductive to heart attacks and strokes. Avoiding omega-6 is the hip thing and healthy thing.

Gut leaky foods

Leaky guts let into the circulation millions of antigens (foreign bodies), and caused eventual inflammatory states in the body (see chapter one for details). Some foods can easily cause the leaky gut syndrome. These foods are to be avoided: Wheat and flour products, too much beans and legumes, kidney beans, soybeans, peanuts, alcohol, hot chili-peppers, milk, nightshade proteins from foods like eggplants, tomatoes, potatoes, and cayenne peppers. High dose of high fructose corn syrups can cause leaky gut syndromes too. So is high amount of sugar itself.

But any foods that caused diarrhea in me, I avoid them as if they cause leaky gut syndrome.

Wheat – Most people know wheat contains gluten that can cause the guts to be leaky, ended up compromising the immune system seriously. But there are several other bad things about wheat people seldom know. The worst of it is that it contains a starch that pus fat right on our belly, not a good thing. It can bind away minerals from our foods in the stomach, and it has a carbohydrate called pectin that can coat our intestine preventing nutrient absorption.

To me, its gluten causing leaky gut syndrome is enough for me to stay away from it as much as I can. Yes, the hot Italian and French breads are hard to resist. But I try to eat just a little.

MSG – Monosodium glutamate is the amino acid that makes foods taste good. It is well known because it caused tingling and heat down the spine of sensitive people in Chinese restaurants. Blinded studies denied such occurrence. Most restaurants use it in the world, not only Chinese restaurants. Scientifically some people even tried to say it has a lot of nutritional values.

But the greatest harm it does is perhaps it makes foods taste good. It makes you overeat easily and get fat. You might deny it (I do), but the mice in the laboratory proved it. Mice ate 40% more food when MSG is added to mouse-feed. So MSG makes even mouse-feed taste good. So there may be some genteel mice-gourmets with bow-ties etc.

Many studies were done showing MSG is safe for customary consumption. It would tend to make us fat, that's all. And that is bad enough.

Antibiotic in animal farms – When one animal is sick, all the farm animals gets the antibiotic. Thus is the custom for most farms. The animals grow faster on antibiotics.

Hormones in farm animals – Growth hormones are used to increase milk production in milk-cows (By 15%). Estrogen is used to increase weight in meat cows, but increase fat more than lean meat. There are concerns with these hormones in the beef we eat. They are concentrated in fatty tissues including milk fat.

Saturated fats (not a mistake, just another bad quality of it) — Whatever the environmental toxins there is, the fatty tissues soak them up. These include antibiotics, hormones, pesticides, industrial chemicals, dioxins. It is estimated 1% of dioxin present in the blood is equal to ten times the risk of cancer. So saturated fat is virtually a waste-dump. I certainly don't want to eat too much saturated fats or cheese and make myself one huge garbage-dump.

HFCS — High fructose corn syrup or another new product simply labeled "fructose" are simply lots of sugar, they go to the liver quicker than regular sugar. The liver turns them into fats and fats come out of the liver cells. When this fat could not circulate away quick, they deposit right on the liver. HFCS is thought to be the main cause of the sky-rocketing incidence of "fatty liver disease". HFCS is present in all the processed foods. Fatty liver disease can lead to liver cancer or death when advanced.

Tuft University has one study showing most Americans get more daily calories from HFCS than any other food ingredients. It's time to read labels and not to buy HFCS foods. A new HFCS is simply labeled as fructose.

Starchy foods — It has three times the calories than other similar foods. It is a major reason for dental cavities. It contains fewer antioxidants than other vegetables. High starchy foods include white potato, sweet potato, rice, grains, beans, and pasta. It is easier to keep slim by avoiding starchy foods.

Alcohols — One drink a day, may decrease the chance of fatty liver disease (and heart disease) according to studies. But that's the only good thing. Two drinks a day, our body decreases burning fat. We get fat. Three drinks a day, ladies, chance of (hormone positive) breast cancer increases. Why, it releases estrogen which is one of the causes for breast cancer. It probably does not help people with ED when it releases estrogen.

Sugar causes inflammation — Three studies showed sugar increase internal inflammations:

1. 29 subjects given one can of soda everyday for 21 days. Each can of soda contain 40 grams of sugar. Blood test showed by the 21th day, the fasting blood sugar increased. The bad cholesterol LDL increased. The blood test for inflammation increased too. (The test for inflammation is called CRP).
2. HFCS given to experimental volunteers at 50 gm of sugar, in 30 minutes, blood test showed CRP increased, i.e. inflammation starts.
3. Obese volunteers given one can of soda with regular sugar. Six months later, they developed insulin resistance (on the way to be a diabetic). Both insulin resistance and diabetes is associated with internal inflammations.

Vitamin E "overdose" – High dose vitamin E was thought to be good in the recent past. So a lot of studies were done on mega-dose vitamin E in "golden studies". Several bad things were observed. It could cause neurotoxicity. It was found to increase the incidence of prostate cancer. And it increased the incidence of bleeding strokes. Normal daily requirement for vitamin E is about 200 IU (international units), but those studies were using 2000 IU.

Two things are not right here: One is the dose is too high. The other one is, vitamin E was given to people without deficiency. Both high dose and superfluous supplementation is bad. It leads to bleeding strokes and cancer as proven by those golden studies whose findings are reliable.

On the other hand, if patients are deficient in vitamin E, given high dose may be beneficial. One example was study in Lin Xian. It is a 20 mile square area in central China. One in four people die of cancer of the esophagus, 100 times the average. It was found to be an under-nutrition problem. Old studies showed supplemented with vitamins including vitamin E cut down the death rate from esophagus cancers. Supplement is good when there is deficiency.

Supplement is good when there is the need for it, even if it is given in mega-dose.

In two studies on Alzheimer's Diseases, High dose vitamin E around 2000 IU was found to delay the disease progression by six and seven months. So far, no conventional medicine can achieve that yet. High dose vitamin E is good when needed.

In fact, any vitamins taken at high dose for a long time has its own dangerous effects on health or even survival. It is absolutely important not to take mega-dose of vitamins or herbs.

Trans fat – Diets with trans fats increases the risk of colon cancers. Where can we see trans fats? Most restaurants are still using trans fats. Even in the few states that ban the use of trans fats in food manufacturers, the restaurants are kind of exempted. I always try to avoid eating greasy foods in restaurants. It messed up cholesterols. Like HFCS, it increases inflammations , is suspected as the main cause of metabolic syndrome (over-weight, diabetes, hypertension, and bad cholesterol), There is a report in a respected journal (NEJM – New England Journal of Medicine) that says eating as little as 20 to 60 calories from trans fats, the damage to the body starts. That is the amount of eating just a few cookies that is made with trans fat to enhance the taste, not to say greasy foods in restaurants.

Inflammation causing foods – These foods include dairy, sugar, gluten, salt, sweet foods , i.e. high glycemic index (GI) foods that are sweet and become sugar quick after eating. Low glycemic index fruits become high glycemic index fruits when ripen fully.

High GI foods – Bananas, ice-creams, bread, white bread, white flour, potato chips, white flour products, potatoes, raisins, alcoholic beverages, white rice, and refined grains. They turn into sugar readily.

Bad fats – examples are high omega-6 foods in refined vegetable oils of sun flower, safflower, soybeans and sunflower oils. Trans fats and saturated fats included.

Farm animals – Has ten times more saturated fat than wild animals. Are we supposed to catch wild animals if want meat? No need to, there are bison meat and grass-fed beef that are better than regular farm meats, lower in saturated fats.

Sugar – How bad can sugar be? It is a poison that tastes sweet and good. Just read on.

1. After consuming sugar, it makes one feel sleepy because when there is high sugar in the brain, the dopamine becomes low. Dopamine keeps us alert.
2. It shortens the telomere. Telomere is the tail of the gene-complex we have in the cells. The longer it is, the longer we may live.
3. It is the only fuel cancer cells can grow on. No extra sugar, no cancer cell-grow. I never forget what a night of nutrition including high sugar could do to cancer. One of my patients underwent tough chemotherapy that needed to be given in the hospital. She wanted to soften her liver cancer so she could live longer at least till all her relatives could come from all over the world to visit. The liver cancer became so soft I could not feel them anymore after chemotherapy in the hospital. One night of intravenous nutrition that has high sugar in it. The liver cancer grew back rock-hard. I almost cried, after examining the patient.
4. Bad gut bacteria thrive on sugar. It would be bad news for our health when that happens. This suggests bad gut-bugs "moved in" after foods available from the agricultural revolutions, sugar is one and the others are foods like grains, wheat, milk, and salt.
5. Excessive intake of sugar can cause leaky gut syndrome which will greatly compromise the immune system.
6. Sugar supplies the stuff for bad glycation-end-products (GEP) to form in our blood. This GEP, like inflammation is associated with all chronic diseases.
7. Sugar, if at high level in the blood, can generate free radicals which can hurt any tissues or organs.
8. Eating too much sugar makes us obese, and bad bacteria thrive on it and cause cavities in the teeth.
9. It gives me toothaches, bad ones, after eating foods with sugar and not brushing teeth right away.

High glycemic index (GI) foods are inflammatory – These are sweet-tasting foods and fruits. They turn into sugars very readily, consider them bad foods. These include all ripen fruits, ice cream, bananas, white bread, all white flour products, potato, raisins, white rice, potato chips, alcoholic beverages, crackers, all raisins, all beans except kidney beans. Or any food that is very sweet. Oat meals or cooked but cooled rice are not high GI foods.

White rice is high GI food, it is bad, but not anymore if cooled and mildly reheated. Why? Because of resistant-starch which is a good food, though it has three times the calorie.
Cooked rice cooled in the refrigerator generates resistance starch that is not digested and not turning into quick sugar. In fact, the good bacteria in the gut turned it into short chain fatty acids like butyrate. The surface cells of the gut wall use butyrate as an energy source for gut cells renewal and repair.

Another bad thing about omega-6, a bad fat – It can oxidize LDL cholesterol. White blood cells (WBC) had to get rid of this bad LDL by eating it. But then the WBC attaches to vessel wall and starts plaque formation. This can happen even the cholesterol level is normal. So now it is recognized lowering cholesterol has not decrease the cardiovascular disease. This is recognized by the government and all the health authorities and societies in the world.
But lowering inflammation has proven to lower heart attack chance by the golden study called CANTOS study.

Another thing wheat is bad – It has a chemical called amylopectin. This amylopectin likes to stuff fats in our bellies. Some called it wheat-belly. But beers have a lot of "wheat" in it, so the big belly is also called beer-belly.
In the past, having a big belly used to be a sigh of being well-off and a sign of prosperity for the individuals in old China, just not nowadays, not anywhere in the world. Even though my belly is very small, I still hate it.

High dose antioxidants – cancel out the benefits of exercise. More information of antioxidant overdose can be found in chapter 18.

Trans fat and FDA – In the years 2013, trans fats got dropped out of the list of foods deemed "possibly safe to eat". So trans fat is possibly no longer safe to eat. Is it safe?

1. Trans fat = belly fat
2. Trans fat = increased risk of colon cancers
3. Trans fat = increased precancerous colon polyps
4. Trans fat = increased risk of breast cancers
5. Trans fat = increased chance of heart attack
6. Trans fat = increased chance of stroke
7. Trans fat = increased my chance of food-related diarrheas. The list can go on….

Omega-3(good fat) deficiency – is in 90% of the population. In omega-3 deficiency, eating saturated fat would cause inflammation.

Red meats may not be the problem of heart disease? Lack of fibers is:

Meat eaters eating red meats with lots of fibers have the same cardiovascular risk as vegans (who don't eat red meats). I only consume red meat rarely no matter what the studies said. And I routinely eat a lot of fibers.

Grains and refined carbohydrates – are counted as sugars if one has diabetes. Refined carbohydrates are white rice and white flour made foods. When I eat them, I feel sleepy. Since I have diabetes, a little sugar eaten would make me sleepy almost right away. Why? When my brain is bombarded with high level of sugar, the dopamine level would drop. Dopamine is what keeps me awake and alert.

BBQ food with crispy skins – yes, I'm going to take that away from you. Not to eat it myself, but to peel the crispy skin off for you. The crispy crunchy skin now has polycyclic aromatic hydrocarbons, and heterocyclic amines. They can increase the risk of cancers. Grilled vegetables have the same cancer causing things. If I eat those foods, like on 4th of July, I would eat a lot of fibers to bind the carcinogens (cancer causing stuff) away. And eat some high vitamin C foods or take a vitamin C pill which may neutralize the carcinogens. And the fibers would be food for good gut bacteria that can break down those carcinogens too. But if the skin is too burnt, I would give up eating it.

I generally avoid cooking with high heat. It can generate the carcinogens mentioned above and spoil some nutrition in the foods.

Omega-6 fats – can harm the good gut bacteria. Vegetable oils are rich in omega-6 like corn oil, canola oil, soybean oil, sun flower oil, safflower oil and peanut oils.

All ripen fruits – are quick sugar source. I dare only eat a small piece or two before it makes me sleepy.

Undermining health – by harming gut bacteria are bad foods like gluten-wheat products, sugar and omega-6 fats.

Starchy carbohydrates – beets, parsnips, pumpkins, sweet potatoes, turnips, cooked carrots, winter squash, potatoes, rice, beans legumes, sweet squash, yams, grains etc.

Absolute avoidance if possible – As a last reminder: sugar and sugary foods, processed foods, trans fats, saturated fats and salt and the classical avoidance foods – wheat products like bread (yes, an ordinary piece of white bread has up to 3 grams of sugar, that's what is bad about refined carbohydrates or processed foods), cakes, cookies; milk and cheese.

Good foods - Good foods can make people smarter, build better immune system and looking younger, and 7 to 10 lbs lighter, and more, said repeatedly in this book:

The items mentioned are not in any special order, the idea is to learn them at random repeatedly for the same item for different qualities. I think that makes it easier to remember and more fun to learn, you never know what item is going to be next:

Multivitamin – It is difficult to eat large amount of different foods so we can get enough vitamins. Too many foods eaten will give us obesity. So it is every guru's and every health practitioner's recommendation to take a multivitamin tablet every day. In addition, I take regular dose vitamin D every day since it was low in my blood. Low vitamin D is common in about half of the populations especially people who live in the northern latitudes (in the North). I take additional vitamin C and E at regular dose every other days or less. High dose vitamins/herbs/supplements can be dangerous. It is not something I would do lightly.

Inulin – is a fiber found in foods like garlic, leeks, onions. Good gut bugs love it. In turn they can make you a different individual. Fibers called pectin in apples has even been proven to defeat some cancers.

Fiber-rich foods – It lowers inflammation markers like IL-6, TNF, though CRP remains the same. CPR is not a sensitive test item for inflammation. A new version of CPR called high- sensitivity C-reactive protein (hsCPR) is now available.

Resistant starch – Digested by gut bacteria to become butyrate that heals leaky guts. Healing leaky guts treated all chronic diseases mentioned in this book. They can be found in grains, seeds, legumes, green peas, unripe bananas, apples, sea weed and reheated cooked rice as well as warmly reheated potatoes. These foods are turned into short chain fatty acids like butyrate. Then the mucosal (surface) cells of the gut can use it as energy for repairs or renewal. Just don't overeat.

Fiber contents: If the fiber contents of commercial fiber-capsules are at basic unit of 1 (Weight compared to weight), then the fruits has 2 units, and the vegetables have 8 units. So to match the daily requirement of fibers of more than 40 grams per day, we need to swallow about six dozen capsules. Yet half a plate of cooked non-starchy vegetables is about enough when three meals are added together for calculations.

Sour foods act as fibers too, that include sour dough.

Omega-3 – This good oil is anti-inflammatory. It can be found in fish oil, fatty fish, and similar good oils, mono-unsaturated fatty acids (MUFA) in nuts, seeds, avocadoes, dark chocolate, coconut oils, and duck oils too. Omega-3 can turn on our genes for fat-burning, it helps to lose weight or keep the same weight and curbs the expansion of our abdominal girth.

Anti-inflammatory foods – Include green tea, ginger, quercetin, turmeric, cocoa, avocadoes, and all probiotics.

Coconut oils – It is a good oil. It is anti-inflammatory, lowering the inflammation marker CRP. It also increases HDL, the good cholesterol. It can readily become energy and can get into mitochondria to help energy (ATP) production. It has medium chain (not long chain) fatty acids that can get converted into short chain fatty acids (SCFA) for gut mucosal cell-repairs. When our dendritic-cells in the gut surface detect the presence of SCFA's, it gives orders to the immune system to switch from the attack mole to peace-mode. And T-suppressors are made instead of T-helper cells (helping to fight wars). The T-cells are one type of the white blood cells. When the T-cells fight wars, it will cause inflammations, local or whole body. So I am cooking with coconut oils. It smells great, and it has high smoking-point so I can use higher temperature if I need to. The next item on coconuts again will give you a secret item of helping erectile dysfunction. Watch for it if you want.

Studies of Omega-3 and unsaturated fats in heart attacks or deaths showed they are **good fats** to eat. In two large studies, they lower the chance of a second heart attack by 70%, and lower the death rate from fatal heart attacks (from second heart attacks) by 45% . These were the Lyon Heart study and the GISSI studies respectively. Those good fats are part of the Mediterranean diets using a lot of fatty fish, olive and olive oils, and strongly vegetable based. Western diet is meat based. Good fats are the mono-unsaturated fats like fatty fish, olive oil, avocado oil, vegetable oils, dark chocolate, duck oil(polyunsaturated fats more) in eating duck meats, walnuts, and macadamia nuts, pecans etc.

How do good fats save lives and the abdominal girth?

Omega-3 and other good fats can switch on the gene for fat

burning and turn off the gene for fat storage. So that in the long run, the abdominal girth may come down (only if you eat 80% full). They can save lives because they lower the internal inflammation in our bodies. This will lower the chance of heart attacks. The above studies in the paragraph immediately above showed the convincing results.

MUFA – are monounsaturated fatty acids. These are very good fats like olive, olive oil, avocado, nuts and seeds. Dark chocolates without sugar are included. They are part of the good fats I used as snacks in between meals when I am really hungry. They last a long time to keep me full. They are the important ingredients to keep my belly so small that it is easily covered up with clothing (I just have to remember eating 80% full, fats gives twice the amount of calories).

Good carbohydrates – Whole foods of carbohydrates are "good-carbs". Non-starchy carbohydrates are good too, so are carbohydrates (vegetables and fruits) that are not sweet. Some examples are cauliflowers, spinach, garlic, onions, leeks, asparagus, cabbage and those green leaves vegetables.

To increase metabolism, burn more fats, and lose weight – is to eat more good proteins, and good fats. GOOD PROTEINS are lean meats, white meats, chicken meat, sea foods, fish meat, crustaceans, shrimps. Avoid big fish meats which have high mercury contents. Or you can eat more GOOD FATS like olive, olive oils, avocados, dark chocolate without added sugars, nuts and seeds. Use coconut oils for cooking, Ok to eat duck meats which are mostly poly-unsaturated fats.

Take high protein diets to lose weight is effective, but cannot be continued for months or years. In the long run, it brings obesity and cardiovascular disease, because proteins mean meats. Meat usually comes with sizable amount of saturated fat. The easy way to lose weight is to eat 80% full and stop and drink a cup of fluid and makes this a habit.

High fat diet, even if it is good fat, is fattening. Fat has almost double the calories of protein or carbohydrates. Because most people do not stop eating till they feel full. That is 120% full when you finally feel full. If it is good fats, may mean 150% overeating. (Because the stomach won't tell the brain it is full until 20 minutes later).

So the best weight loss diet is plant-based diet. But those plants have to be non-starchy, not sugary, and not refined carbohydrates as in cakes, cookies, and all processed foods in the stores. GOOD CARBS are generally WHOLE FOODS and not starchy and have low glycemic index, i.e. not easily turned into sugar. They don't taste sweet.

Medium chain fatty acids – I think this is the one of the items in programs like "eat fat, get thin". Because coconut drink is so convenient, comes in a milk carton. Just pour it out like a cup of milk, and drink. I drink a small cup once or twice a day. This is good fat from coconut milk. It contains lots of medium chain fatty acids (MCFA) or medium chain triglycerides (MCT). Whatever you call it, it is good. But I limit myself to only a small cup because it has high calories. Too much of it will cause diarrhea in me. Some takes pancreatic enzymes so diarrhea won't happen. But that is unnatural I would hesitate to do.

Medium chain fatty acids (coconut fats in meat and oil)
1.   Medium chain fatty acids like that in coconut oil/milk readily becomes energy and not stored as fat. It would not be picked up by fat cells for deposit like other bad fats such as omega-6 rich foods.
2.   It goes right into mitochondria, the energy factories of cells without any vehicles to take it in necessarily.
3.   When they are in the gut, they are broken down into short chain fatty acids (SCFA). SCFA tells the gut dendritic cells in our body that peace has come, no more wars. The dendritic cells switch on the peace-switch to calm down the immune system, and inflammation comes way down.
4.   They lower anxiety and increase cognition.
5.   It is anti-inflammatory.

International trials of good fats and heart attack or death from heart attacks
1.   Lyon Heart Study – Mediterranean diet vs the American (now infamous) low fat pyramid diet. Mediterranean diet is good fat rich with oils like omega-3, from fatty fish, olive, olive oils, nuts and seeds, and lots of green-leaf veggies. The score? "Meds" win thumbs up. The population of people with hearts

attacks before, now had 70% decrease of a second heart attack. One reason to abandon the "low fat diet" of old time America (only about 5 to 6 decades ago) food pyramid.

2. Another reason to kick the "low fat diet" into infamous history is the GISSI study. The ones with omeg-3 like food won the "super-bowl". They had a 45% drop in fatal (second) heart attacks.

So we can all blame the "low fat diet!" for two to three generations of Americans over-weight or obese with all kinds of chronic diseases! It is all due to the "low fat diet" advice, emphasizing on a lot of carbohydrates but not telling good carbs from bad cards. And then there came the fattening "low fat" diet of processed foods full of calories from HFCS, and trans fats (properly disguised as hydrogenated vegetable oils). And to make the processed foods taste good, there are lots of additives like MSG, fillers, and plenty of salts too. All the HFCS, trans fats and salts are inflammatory. They caused sky high rise of diabetes and obesity.

From now on, I will give a faithful trial of "EAT FAT, GET THIN" diet which is about 60% or higher of non-starchy vegetables and the rest are good fats and some good proteins. I just have to be mindful of the high calorie-density in those good fats.

Legumes – these are beans and peas. Are they good or bad? It depends. They are good in that they have lots of fibers, minerals and vitamins. And they taste good. But on the other hand, they are acid foods. They could decrease vitamin B absorption and cause dry eyes. They also contain lectins. In large amount, lectins could cause leaky gut syndrome like glutens do, in sensitive people. Whether they are good foods or bad foods, the verdict depends on an individual's sensitivities, I think. But they are starchy foods if eaten in large amount. They are bad then when one eats a lot of it.

Benefits of proteins (meats) – High-protein diet is the sure way to lose weight. But it may be harmful if continued long term, especially if the percentage of protein in a meal is more than 35%. One can run into protein toxicity of nausea, vomiting, and sudden loss of weight and feeling sick. Like good fats, good proteins do switch on fat burning and decrease fat storage (at the belly). They both increase the rate of metabolism to burn off more calories faster. If you eat too much protein or good fats, they won't be stored as body fat easily, though you could get fat too, just not as readily. Remember eating till 80% full plus a cup of water to make it feel like 100%

Coconut oil or meat and erectile dysfunction – The oils (medium chains fatty acids) in coconuts promote the conversion of cholesterol to pregnenolone which can be converted to DHEA, which will give you either estrogen or testosterone. In the bodies of elderly male like me, probably low in testosterone, DHEA probably will be converted to testosterone and help with my ED. After starting my plan to follow "EAT FAT, GET THIN" program after reading Mark Hyman, MD's book of the same name, I do feel sex life got more enjoyable. I mainly drink half a cup of coconut drink. I hope this would last and not a placebo effect.

Good fats shut off the hungry center of the brain – This was seen by doing brain imaging. But personally, I find it to be true too. As I began eating more fat, just by drinking a small cup of coconut drink from a container like a milk-carton bought from big store. I stopped needing a nap at noon time. At the same time, I also cut way down on eating starchy carbohydrates like noodles and rice. The small cup of coconut drink has enough calories to replace the carbohydrates I cut out from meals. Too much carbs get people tired, and hungry easily.

Good fats and sex drives etc – good fats make life better, studies has found out that good fats increase energy, increase digestion, mood, joint pain, allergies, and yes, it improves sex drive too, no less. That has been what I have been feeling, all of the above. I achieve this simply by drinking a coconut drink. And in between meals when I am hungry, I chew on a handful of walnuts which are rich in good oils omega-3 compared to inflammatory oils omega-6.

Low carbohydrates benefit – My plate of a meal has 50% area filled with non-starchy cooked vegetables. That amount to about 40% of the total calories at best. 40% carbohydrates meal is low-carb meal. Has there been already fats deposited on my liver though not reaching bad "fatty liver disease" from the infamous "low-fat diet"? But my low fat diet and high carbohydrates diet in the past decades no doubt has created some extra fat and deposited on the liver. Because the excess carbohydrates from past low-fat diets got turned into fats by the liver. And some would have been deposited right in the liver, no doubt. I do not have fatty liver disease because my blood tests for the liver have been normal.

The high fat diet I am adapting to will stop excess carbohydrates being converted by the liver into fats. So I think my liver is going to be less fatty in the future.

This begs the answer to the question:" Does low carbohydrate diet get rid of liver fats?" From studies, the answer is affirmative. "Low carb" diet did prove to "decrease liver fat content". (Please note, not low fat diet but low carb diet). Half a plate of non-starchy vegetables is about 40% carbohydrates, is low carb diet.

Low carbohydrate diet is anti-inflammatory too.

Eggs are good foods – Eggs does raise the LDL level, despite what industry-sponsored studies in the past claimed that it did not per Physician Committee for Responsible Medicine review of the industry-sponsored studies that claimed it did not raise LDL. But it is clear now the "lowering of cholesterol level does not bring less cardiovascular disease". All health authorities, including the government's dietary guideline advisory committee acknowledged that in 2015. So who is going to worry about cholesterol level anymore? If cardiovascular disease is caused by chronic inflammation, and as proven by various huge studies, like the studies of lowering the inflammation with Mediterranean diet as in the Lyon Heart study and the GISSI study, both lowered heart attacks and dying of heart attacks. It's the inflammatory foods, the bad foods, we need to avoid. That should wipe out the worries of eggs increasing LDL anymore. New food-sciences also told us, good fats, even when raising the LDL, it is the harmless bigger fluffy LDL that is raised. Not the small dense LDL that starts the plaques.

Eggs are absolutely the best available source of fats and proteins, vitamins for everything, especially for the eyes because in eggs, there are also the antioxidants Lutein and Zeaxanthine, and all the essential amino acids that we need are there. I am so glad now, that in the past I ate two eggs daily. I thought it was dangerous. It is not dangerous anymore. But I won't eat two eggs every day as it contains a high amount of omega-6, a bad fat that is inflammatory. Eating too many eggs daily could result in increase in internal inflammation.

I insist on buying cage-free eggs. Though as any chicken farmers would have told me, in a chicken farm, is it very hard to be really a 100% "go green".

The good vitamin E can be bad if ... - vitamin E is an antioxidant, and anti-inflammatory. People who take this supplement will see their internal inflammation go down by 30 to 50% as shown in studies. This lowering of inflammation easily decrease nasal allergies. At 200 IU (international units) a day, it was shown to improve the immune system. At 100 IU a day, even the lesions (plaques) in arteries had been shown to go down. This is good, low or regular dose Vit E.

But it can be bad when given at high dose of more than 400 IU a days for years. A study showed people taking more than 400 IU daily had more pre-matured deaths. In "golden studies", such high dose of vitamin E caused increased hemorrhagic strokes, and it fostered the growth of prostate cancers.

High dose vitamins are always dangerous. Evan normal dose of vitamins given to people who are not deficient in that vitamin is dangerous, as some studies showed.

But when one is "deficient" in certain vitamins, mega-dose can be beneficial.

Meg-dose vitamin E delayed Alzheimer's disease progression for six or seven months

For mild or moderate Alzheimer's disease, two golden studies showed the progression of the disease was delayed by 6 and 7 months was possible. The dose of vitamin E given daily was like 2000 IU. That's mega-dose. But in a disease where almost nothing works to delay it, this treatment is a viable option.

Good fat is anti-inflammatory – a good fat called gamma linolenic acid (GLA) is proven anti-inflammatory. In a study of treatment for rheumatoid arthritis (RA) disease, a very inflammatory auto-immune disease (the immune system attacking oneself), GLA given to RA patients for one year, shrank their swollen joints by 40%.

What can anti-inflammatory GLA, vitamin E, and Omega-3 do together? Olympic gold/silver/bronze medals

(Sorry, not for you or me). The Danish rowing team won a lot of Olympic gold medals. I believed it was the year 1996 the supplements mentioned above helped them win the gold medal. In their intense day-long rowing practice preparing for the Olympics, all the crew members over-worked their joints into big time arthritis. The combination of gamma-linolenic acid, omega-3 fish oils, and vitamin E came to their rescue. The joints were totally healed in a month. They were able to continue practicing rowing. Eventually they got themselves the Olympic gold medal. There were a lot more medals to follow thanks to the anti-inflammatory treatments of the supplements and their ingenious work out. NSAD is not going to do it, I strongly suspect.

(I just hope an Olympic champion is not reading this, because I said sorry, not for you or me to the medals).

I only take vitamin E at regular dose 3 times per week

I once had a mild feeling of right calf claudication (pain during exercise) symptoms after running out of supply of *Ginkgo biloba*. So I suspect in the calf arteries, there might be plaque narrowing the blood vessels. And vitamin E is able to decrease plaque lesions, revealed by studies. So I take vitamin E to try to decrease the inflammation that would lead to decrease plaques. But one study showed in deficiency of selenium, a rare mineral, taking vitamin E could increase the chance of prostate cancer. So I avoid taking it every day. And I am taking multi-vitamin that contains selenium, daily.

But how come vitamin E can decrease plaques? In studies, it is found out that vitamin E protects the arteries by preventing smooth muscle proliferation that can narrow the arteries. It also prevents monocytes (white blood cells) adhesion to vessel walls, and platelet (a blood "cell") adhesion is prevented also. Platelets are incorporated as part of the plaque compositions. Vitamin E can cause vessel dilation also in rabbit studies.

What can fibers do for health? — take fibers in the resistant starches for example, it is resistant to our digestion. When resistant

starch is digested by gut bacteria to become butyrate, butyrates supply the energy for the gut cells to mend themselves. That heals the leaky guts. Healing leaky guts treated all chronic diseases mentioned in this book. As stated before in the paragraph listing foods containing resistant starches, warmly reheated previously cooked rice and potatoes contains resistant starches.

Butyrate is a short chain fatty acid. When short chain fatty acids are detected by our dendritic-cells in the gut wall, it give signals to the immune system to stop the immune wars. Immune wars bring tons of inflammatory chemicals. Now peace time comes, the inflammation goes way down. Chronic diseases "cured" when inflammation goes down. This is perhaps the greatest thing fibers can do for our health, to bring peace to the immune system and end chronic diseases.

Besides, fibers can also bind toxins, sugars, cholesterols, bad fats and prevent their absorption to a great degree. It can decrease the risk of colon cancers by various mechanisms.

What foods can lower inflammations besides fibers? – all good proteins, good fats, and low carbohydrate diets can lower internal inflammations in our bodies.

Omega-3 foods – some examples are walnuts, marine fatty fishes like sardines, mackerel, anchovy, salmon, trout, flaxseeds, hemp, chia seeds, olives, coconuts, and cocoa nibs.

Grain-free diets – It decreases schizophrenia symptoms. Grains were not stable foods of mankind in the Old Stone Age people. Yet, the digestive system of mankind had evolved for millions of years without grains. Grains are products of agricultural revolution that happened about 10 thousand years ago. So a lot of people's genes may not have changed enough to digest and handle grains. Then they would be sensitive to grains. In them, eating grains will bring internal inflammations.

Anti-mutagenesis foods – are foods that are against mutations in our genes. Mutation in genes can lead to mutated cells developing cancers. These foods include garlic, ginger, citrus peels, turmeric and burdock. There are 5000 mutations daily in us. Our immune system gets rid of those mutated cells.

Health and immune systems promoting life-styles

Fasting – that includes 500 calories a day as fasting. Two days a week of fasting are good enough, or even one day. The benefits are many:
1. Fasting increases the variety of gut bugs and decrease inflammation.
2. Fasting may restore basic gut bacteria variety which may be the probable most beneficial original combination for our health, mental and physical.
3. The original gut-bacterial composition had restored the basic female hormones combinations in a young woman who had female hormone total-ablation treatment to prevent menstruation so she would not bleed to death during menstruation. Her story can be read in detail in chapter41, one of the cases of spontaneous healing stories, two chapters later.

For clinical fasting book, Dr Mosley's "the FastDiet" is a good read. But in actually doing it, one needs a health professional's guidance for safety. I, on the other hand, need a lot of will-power.

Adequate sleep – Sleep deprivation is the most common reason for stress in America, one study showed. Sleep deprivation leads to the increase of appetite. So we all obese people can blame it on sleep deprivation, right? No! Everyone needs to have six to eight hours of sleep. We need to turn off the TV and get to bed at 10PM or 11PM. Stress brings internal inflammation that brings more than obesity. It also brings diabetes, heart attack, stroke and cancers. Not to say the 33 chronic diseases I had cured by lowering internal inflammation. Sleep deprivations may bring them all back.

At times like this with the Respiratory virus pandemic sweepingly infecting people globally, sleep deprivation came into sharp focus to me, because it weakens the immune systems that led to the deaths of young doctors and nurses who were bombarded with thousands of new patients and had to work day and night. Studies most recently already showed the disease fighting white blood cells called Natural Killer (NK cells) cells decreased by 70% in sleep deprivation. Other white blood cells and cytokines decreased too. NK cells are key virus fighting cells. This is a much weakened immunity even the mild infection, which the Respiratory virus pandemic infection is, could kill. We all need 6 to 8 hours of sleep daily or more.

High intensity exercise training – even 2 minutes of it every week, before we slow-down in whatever exercise we are doing is good enough to boost our metabolism and increase the number of our gut bacteria (That is good, you should believe me by now). This was a paper published in JAMA (Journal of the American Medical Association).

Stress reduction – The most practical way to do that is to lower the internal inflammation. When that task was achieved, my mind was clear of brain fogs, I had no moody times because honestly, my terrible mood-swing as my wife claimed it to be, has all but gone. This achievement is the proudest thing I have done. So I think remember the bad foods and avoid them is the single most important thing to lower my internal inflammation that brings tremendous release of stress and mental strain.

For everything I described in all these chapters, I would not encourage you to do the same things I did, until after running it by a health professional. But for bring this book everywhere to remember the BS in this chapter, I whole-heartedly encourage you to do so. It will probably build a very healthy life for you. The following could relieve stress when practiced. But I still maintain the best way to do it is by avoiding bad foods and eating good foods so the mood can be elevated, stress can just evaporate in the air.

Simple meditation to enlighten the mind

One method of stress reduction I do is meditations when I feel I need one. I close my eyes, pay 100% attention to every detail in my breathing movements of how the muscles move, how the air moves. Even for a few minutes, I would be refreshed.

Meditation could change the anatomy of our brain's structure and function. A study showed those long term meditation people have a different anatomy in the area associated with positive moods, in the left prefrontal cortex (around the temporal areas in the brain), it affects attention and learning.

There are quite a few studies suggesting release stress, the habit of meditation with deep breathing and concentrating the attention on the mechanics of deep breathing is very effective, and simple to do. Sometimes repeating certain numbers in my mind helps.

Other benefits of reducing stress

1. Good hormones goes up, bad hormones go down, life is better.
2. Testosterones goes up, sex life may be enhanced
3. Stress weight gain is around the belly, I look forwards to finishing this book, so my abdominal girth may go down (writing a good book could be stressful) with the release of stress. Look forward to a life with less stress and lots of fishing. But to be honest, I have derived great pride and pleasure in being able to collect so much beneficial statements and share it with my readers.
4. Once again, it is a delight to mention, inflammation goes down as the blood test for inflammation would go down too as stress is relieved.

To have no want so we won't feel being deprived and all stressed out. Just the thought of it is like hearing a clear silver-bell ding in the air.

Another good way to reduce stress is psychological. I truly believe in Confucian and Tao philosophy of looking at the material world as what it is, enough is as good as gold. Some philosophers would say, "To have no want". This is very important because when we watch TV, all the advertisements would poison our mind to have things that we don't really need, but the convincing ads all tell us to "want it, got to have it". The feeling of being deprived of something spring right into our minds and is very poisoning. It raises our stress inside without us knowing it, because most of the time, in the real world, those are things we probably cannot afford and yet we don't really need.

Therefore makes it simple for our lives, always remember the spirit of "to have no want" and "enough is as good as gold", especially when those beautiful advertisement comes on. It's good just to admire the advertisements like a beautifully done piece of art and nothing else.

Some necessary vitamins – There is no way I can get all the vitamins in foods I eat. There are too many minerals and vitamins that are lacking in foods I usually eat. I think that applies to everyone. Because the soil from which all the foods grow is severely depleted of nutrients and minerals. So I take a multivitamin daily. For most elderly people, vitamin D and calcium is not enough from the foods we eat. But all vitamins have to be taken at regular dose, and only take when there is a deficiency.

Some examples of food contaminants – Avoid eating them is a very important healthy life-style.

.Fatty meats – all hormones used by farmers, and toxins in the environment can be dissolved in fat. Like estrogen that make cattle make more fatty meat, synthetic growth hormones for producing more milk. These hormones make you fat. And the concentrated estrogens in cheese have been associated with 49% more deaths from patients with breast cancers who were cured of breast cancers but consumed more than one serving of cheese daily from a recent study.

.Environmental toxins got concentrated in fats too. They are a main suspect for increasing inflammation and increase in chronic diseases over the past couple of decades: Acnes, asthmas, obesity, diabetes, allergies and more. The increases are generally described as astronomical.

.All processed foods when analyzed by their constituents are almost the same. They are lots of sugar, fat, salt, MSG, coloring, fillers plus a little bit of the real food. Besides this little bit of real food, sometimes as little as 10%, all other additives that make up the food are "contaminants".

Processed foods

All processed foods are made with one goal in the maker's mind, to make it tasty to hook you up, whatever material they have to use. The food conferences are just discussions and exchange of experience of how to hook you up, I refused to be a sucker, given in to a tasty food to bring inflammation back and along comes with all the 33 chronic disease. These are mainly the processed foods in the stores, not the whole foods.

Omega-3 (good oil) to Omega-6 (bad oil) ratio in nuts

Not all nuts are created equal to the good fats (omega-3) to bad fats (omega-6) ratios. Only walnuts, macadamian nuts and pecans have decent good fats to bad fats ratios. Most other nuts have very high omega-6 contents. Though they have plenty of protein, minerals and vitamins making them good foods too, but just a handful to eat is good enough. More of it is harmful (too many calories) and may be inflammatory.

Is taking probiotics good? See their functions for us -

Probiotics refers to the bacteria mainly in our colon. More scientific evidence points to these trillions of bacteria in our gut as just another organ for us. Collectively, their weight is 3 to 5 pounds. They have genes numbering 4 million, compared to human genes of 23,000. What is unique in bacterial DNA is that scientific analysis showed most of the bacterial genes are for some function or some structures that influence human cell functions. There is not a day in Google News without mentioning new findings about the gut bacteria related to our health.

Every health guru's book emphasizes foods with a lot of fibers just for these bacteria. Fibers are their foods. They turn the fibers into energy our colonic mucosal cells (The surface cells in the colon) can use as energy for maintenance and repair.

We can just take a glance at what this bacterial human-organ can do, then you know, their mere existence is for our survival, so they can seed our descendants' guts when the newborns pass through the vaginal canal and swallow a mouthful of them into their baby colons. So that when we survive, they survive. They evolved for millions of years to just to work collectively as a human organ. It seems to me, it is their honor to work for us and they are all welcome guests.

So I got to forget what I learned in medical school about bacteria. That was: what is the best antibiotic to kill them. Surely, for some of these bacteria that got in the wrong place of our body and cause infection, the old medical knowledge of antibiotics is still essential.(Like the skin bacteria in our blood causing fever, we need to kill them still with very strong antibiotics). But for those guest bacteria in the right place in our colon, I would use a lot of fibers to welcome them, to please them.

Without them, our immune system would not mature and function as it is supposed to be. In the mice devoid of gut bacteria, because they are raised in a sterile environment, eat sterile foods, breath sterile air. (A lot of scientific experiments depend on them). But these mice, without bugs in their guts, their immune system does not mature nor would it protect them against infections. One infection, they are going to die.

1. Besides, these specially grown mice called nude mice (without hair) don't have vitamin K to start blood clotting. Once they bleed, they can bleed to death. We are not much better than the mice with respect to making vitamin K, we don't make vitamin K also, though we've got vitamin K in our blood to stop bleeding. The bacteria in our gut make the vitamin K for us, otherwise, we have no vitamin K (vitamin K is hundreds of other hormones and other molecules they make for us). I think this point well-illustrates the function of the bacterial human-organ.

2. But this bacterial human-organ is a dynamic one. We eat the wrong foods can make them change their population composition. That is why there are good foods, and there are bad foods. The bad foods we mentioned so far would give us bad bugs.

   A clinical case would illustrate the difference between fat-oriented and slim oriented bacterial human-organ combination. (A fat lady has a fat-oriented combination of bacteria, while a thin lady has a slim-oriented combination of bacteria in the colons).

   There was a clinical case every fecal transplant physicians knows. Fecal transplant is filtering the stool and get the bacteria into water, and either use a tube up the colon to deposit the bacteria combination there or take a capsule of bugs. This is fecal transplant. This clinical case involved a slim mother who was treated with antibiotic for an infection. She developed the antibiotic induced diarrhea. No drug worked to stop the diarrhea. Death could ensure soon. So the fecal water with combination of bacteria in it from her daughter was used for the fecal-transplant to cure the fatal diarrhea. Her daughter was obese. The bacterial combination was fat-oriented.

The slim mom got the fecal transplant from her daughter. The dangerous diarrhea stopped. Before long, the slim mom's became obese fast from then on. Now fecal transplant physicians make sure the donor is not obese. But we cannot treat obesity by fecal transplant, as only life-threatening disease would warrant a fecal transplant for now. There are still a lot of unknowns about this treatment. One case recently of a man receiving fecal transplant ended up dying of it. This tells us, only life-threatening cases warrant this treatment till more is leaned about the gut bacteria in fecal transplant.

3. Do you believe our brain cells may need the help of gut bacteria to make new brain cells? In a mice experiment, the new brain cells are labeled. So you can tell which cells are new cells by the labeling chemicals. The mice were then given strong antibiotic, and kill a lot of the gut bacteria. The new brain cells stopped being made when the mice's gut- bacteria is eradicated by antibiotics. So just these few examples showed us how intimately the bacterial human-organ has evolved to serve us. There is a chapter on them being a chemical factory for us next in chapter 40. But remember the bugs even is related to making brain cells for the host, then you know the importance of foods with a lot of fibers, the non-starchy vegetables,

Currently, taking commercial probiotics are indicated for irritable bowel syndrome, Crohn's disease, intractable diarrhea, and ulcerative colitis. Taking it for health reasons may not have been so well worked out yet. But so far taking commercial preparation has not seen bad side effects, though they could cause stomach upsets, bloating, gas, constipation etc. But we take it at our own risk. Though in the case of the fatal fecal transplant, there was an antibiotic resistant bacteria that was transplanted and cause fatal infection. Might be, the host only had a weak immune system. So I would worry if an individual is weak in his or her immune system, whether it is safe to take probiotics or not? So far there is no answer.

Exercise is an important good life-style – Exercise makes me feel happy, that's why I kept on swimming. In fact, my right shoulder and right knee joints' function depends on it also. So I will never stop exercising. In addition to the personal reasons, I am going to code a couple of studies to say it even can control cancer.

1. In the Nurses Health Study, a hundred million dollar study (the cost is to show its importance) it showed rigorous exercise vs regular exercises make a difference in the colon cancer occurring. The rigorous exercise group has 50% less colon cancer.

2. In fact, from my past data collection for my other 3 books, exercise prevent 40% of cancers, prevent 50% recurrence, and decrease deaths from cancer by yes, the same 50% as a general statement.

3. New sciences finding of benefits of exercises, however, add spice to the already good reports (Thousands of positive reports). It may make us live longer. It lengthened the tail of the gene-complex (telomeres) by 9 years. Do you want 9 more years to live? If you do, make sure you physically can do it, be cleared by your own physician so you can do high level of exercises (18 METS). That is equal to fast running for a little more than two solid hours, or swimming pretty quickly for 3 hours per week. (I think I may get that 9 more years). For slow walking, it takes 8 hours, rope jumping is 1.8 hours per week.

To sum up –

This is a big chapter trying to include all modern sciences findings of foods and life-style and how it affects our health and well-being. I called it beneficial statements, abbreviated BS, to show it is not BS in its conventional sense (Which means garbage), but that these are real beneficial statements (BS). The abbreviation "BS" would easily remind readers to read it whenever there is time, I hope, so their health can be better. And chronic diseases can be cured.

You can see there are so much new studies and findings about good foods, bad foods and good life-styles. There are 32 pages of the BS or so. It is a lot of good information (about 90 main points). But take the book along for doctor's visits, for your vacation just to see what new sciences have been found. Repeated reading is a necessity for this chapter so you can rip the benefits of these food and life-style sciences. These sciences are new and so may be hard to digest. But repeated reading and comprehension will lead one to a better world. Of all the things I learned in life, these BS are the best.

In time, your health information gained probably may benefit you like what they have benefited me. But make sure to consult your own health care professional before taking up things I have done. As a medical doctor, I feel this is the appropriate thing to do, so it can be safe for you. But after knowing the information well, you know how to choose good foods, avoiding bad foods. Can you do it on your own? Yes if you know you have no sensitivity to those foods.

When you start eating it more, your taste bud will grow to like it in two weeks. Even if it is good foods, like sea-foods, can cause fatal allergy in the sensitive individuals. Allergy tests in a doctor's office can reveal if you are allergic to any new foods you have not tried before.

But for herbal medications, or even simple vitamins or other supplements, it does need a knowledgeable professional to check for drug interactions, contra-indications, to make sure it is safe for you. For endurance exercise and high intensity exercises, most of us would need a doctor's evaluation and see if we are fit to do it.

Enjoy a good healthy life. Best wishes.

Chapter Forty - Evidence of gut bacteria (microbiome) collectively works as a chemical factory for us

Most gut bacterial genes evolved to make molecules for human

There are trillions of gut bacteria weighing 3 to 5 pounds in our colon. They have 4 millions genes. Humans have 23 thousands genes only. What functions do most of the huge numbers of bacterial genes serve? Most bacterial genes, on analysis, are found to "make molecules that can affect human cell functions". Are they trying to take over by affecting our cell functions the way scientists put it? No. Those bacterial molecules are to be modified by us for our own use.

Looks like the bacteria in our guts have evolved to make chemicals for us. Every day in Google News, there is one more human function made possible by gut bacteria. So the scientific discovery about gut bacterial function for us is being found every day. In this chapter, I would just describe some chemicals the scientists have already found that are made by the gut bacteria for human use. In the last chapter, we have seen vitamin K is made by bacteria for us, or for their hosts, the laboratory mice. So blood-clotting in humans and mice can happen. So wounds can stop bleeding.

And the immune system of ours and the mice depend on gut bacteria for maturation and proper function. And at least in mice, the making of brain cells depended on gut bacteria. Only God knows how many chemicals they made to achieve maturation of the immune system and making brain cells.

In this chapter, I am just going to list the functions or chemicals the gut bacteria made for us. From these data, I got the feeling that the bacteria in our gut has evolved to serve us as a chemical factory. Why? Because only if our ancestors survive, then the gut bugs in our ancestors survive. So they had to help the life of our ancestors by making good chemicals for them. What chemicals?

1. Bacteria made happy hormones for us, so we feel alright. First one is dopamine, 40% made in China or USA? No, neither. This is made in the bacteria working like "human-organ" in our gut, absorbed by us for our own happiness.

2. 90% of our serotonin, another happy hormone, is made by bacteria for our use.

3. Klebsiella, a common bacteria, can make B12 and vitamin K. We gladly absorb them and use them. By the way, we don't have the genes to make vitamin K or B12, two very necessary vitamins to make sure if we bleed, clots will form and that our nerve and brain functions can be maintained respectively. So we won't bleed without stopping till death shall come, the function of vitamin K, or be anemic and crazy, the function of B12.

4. Gut bacteria help digest carbohydrates for us. There are quite a few enzymes involved in this digestion of the carbohydrates, probably some enzymes are made by bacteria, used by us.

5. The bacteria Akkermansia is associated with slimness in us. I just wish I know what chemical is involved. That would be worth of a Nobel Price, right?

6. When we eat more fibers, including fibers from resistant starch, bacteria turn the fibers into short chain fatty acids (SCFA) like butyrate. Butyrate is the energy source for mucosal cells (surface cells) of the gut to do maintenance job and repair of our gut wall. The presence of the SCFA in the gut signals our mucosal dendritic cells to switch on the peace-and-no-war mode. Without the gut bugs, we probably never can operate our immune system. What to do in peace mode? Maintenance.

7. The same SCFA are signals for our dendritic cells to turn the immune system into peace mode, making T-suppressor cells, and making other immune cells stop making chemicals of inflammation. Our systemic inflammation is over. That is the function of the chemical butyrate made by gut bacteria.

8. Gut bacteria can prevent cancer in mice which are destined to have colon cancer. These mice have their IL-10 gene knocked-out for the holy search of knowledge. They will develop colon cancer. But if these mice are given probiotics containing a few good gut bacteria, presumably making IL-10 for them, cancer won't happen. God bless those scientists and those bacteria. Members of the families with hereditary gut disease that predispose to colon cancers may someday prevent their colon cancers by taking those good bacteria capsules. Then they may not have to have their colons preventively removed, and lead a

very inconvenient life. But that needs research.

9. To protect the colon against cancers in us, gut bacteria can break down carcinogens or produce chemicals like butyrate to repair our injured gut cells so cancer won't happen in the injured cells which is normal after repair.

10. Another strain of mice is destined to have bladder cancers. But if they drink fermented milk containing good gut bacteria, some lucky mice can avoid bladder cancers. The same finding was reported in human studies also. That suggested the immune system is strengthened by the bacteria in mice and humans.

11. Sometimes, some harmful bacteria like E. coli, Enterococcus, or Salmonella may want to establish colonies in our colon. But the good bugs have chemicals to stop them from doing that. If these bad bugs take over, it is the end of us.

12. There was an interesting control study that was randomized and double blinded, and proved beyond doubt that taking probiotics can prevent "calling in sick" days from work. This happened in a company in Sweden in the year 2005.

    181 of their workers were given a drink to go with lunch. Half were given just the drink. The other half had the same drink with probiotics coating the straws. Eighty days later, there were 26 called in sick workers in the control group, while in the probiotic group, there were only 16 call in sick workers. So it is obviously suggesting once again, the bacteria enhanced the immune system so less people called in sick.

To sum up –

It is looking more and more likely the three to five pounds of bacteria in our colon has evolved to work like a chemical factory for us, making B12, vitamin K, dopamine, serotonoin, IL-10, and butyrate. This I did not include the other new agents and functions scientists found and reported in Google news every week. The Bcteria even has a role in making brain cells, avoiding cancers, keeping people from calling in sick.

It is legitimately a bacterial human-organ. Huh? So what shall we call it? What? Wait a minute, whoa, you want to call it "Mutiny on the Bounty"?

Chapter Forty One - Cases and Sciences of spontaneous Healings including Cancers.

Sciences of spontaneous healing – The sciences are very simple. It is the theme in this book. "Avoid bad foods to heal the gut, to restore the natural immune-system plus smart life-styles, it will get rid of the chronic diseases". That is it. This is the basic science that made all these cases of spontaneous healings. The 33 chronic diseases of mine I got rid off are real examples of so called spontaneous healings too.

In the first place, when I had those 33 chronic diseases, the immune system was busily fighting a "world war". There was infection-like fighting all over my body. It was not real infection. But the immune system was presented with bacterial parts in the blood all over my body. These bacterial parts leaked into my system from the gut, as we have learned throughout the book. I had irritable bowel syndrome. My immune cells were greatly "outnumbered" or "Beyond capacity to function" and my immune system slid into chaos. "Not a good thing".

The immune system was evolved to handle local wars, like focal infections on wounds of the skin. Let's call these local wars. But if the infection is all over the body, the individuals died often. (We are calling this whole body infection as a "world war"). That happened in the old days before antibiotics. Now, with antibiotics for bacterial infections, most people will get to live when the infection is in the blood, all over the body. (A lot of people still die of this world war like whole body infection by bacteria in the blood -- bacteremia).

But modern medicine is still in its infancy of trying to cure viral infections. A viral infection all over the body can easily be fatal. The immune system has no capacity to fight them. It will only get out of control. That is why with the viral infection called Ebola, 50% of the people dies. This is just because the human immune system was evolved only to fight focal wars, not world wars (like infection all over the body).

The leaky gut syndrome of mine let in millions of dead bacterial parts from my gut. My immune system fights them but could not handle this "world war" situation. It was not only greatly weakened, it ran out of control, attacking my guts to keep the irritable syndrome, attacking my joints for the arthritis, attacking my nose and throat to keep the allergy, (that I needed to take Zyrtec daily for allergy). For the same reason, the body was under attack everywhere, all my chronic diseases happened, 33 chronic diseases in all. Till I healed my gut by avoiding bad foods, the "world war" was over. My now quiet immune system stopped its attack on my body, and all the chronic diseases disappeared. This quiet down immune system can even get rid of cancers as we will see later in this chapter in three examples of cancers spontaneously resolved.

This is the science of spontaneous healing. It is done by restoring the immune system so it can function properly in the background of living healthy life-styles. Then cancers went away; Rheumatoid arthritis cured, and a 10 year old boy came out of steroids; disabling muscle inflammation gone (myositis); even autism patients cured; as well as infertility and bone marrow failure (aplastic anemia) in a young lady who failed bone marrow transplant twice, cured, and her infertility due to treatment, eventually cured so she could give birth to four children in 20 years. All this happened by eating good foods healing the gut.

Avoiding bad foods to heal the gut, spontaneous healings happened. This is the simple basic sciences in all these cases. So now let's see the miracles of life reported by different health gurus.

Spontaneous healing cases 1, 2, and 3 – cancers

Case one is still in the internet of a 3 years old called Molly with right eye Kaposi's sarcoma (6). It is a deadly cancer in her age-group. It was clinically diagnosed. Parents refused biopsy. But the case was presented in Opthalmology grand-round and published publicly. The diagnosis was sure clinically, even without biopsy. After diagnosis, Molly was found to also have celiac disease, much like an irritable bowel syndrome. She was allergic to gluten that caused celiac disease. One week after avoiding gluten containing foods, the ophthalmologist could see the cancer was getting smaller. Two months into the gluten free diet, the Kaposi's sarcoma totally disappeared. The case is still on line.

I typed in the words "3 years old Molly with Kaposi's sarcoma" on Google Search, I still could retrieve the case history and see the clear pictures of the cancer disappearing from Molly's eyes. I first saw those pictures in Tom O'Bryans, DC. CCN, DAC, BN 's book (6).

Case # 2 was my own patient from years ago (36, 37,38). She was a middle age lady with carcinoid tumor (low grade cancer) in her left lower lung near the spine. It was a golf ball size mild cancer (Sometimes it can be fatal fast). Usually surgery is not a commonly recommended choice in this mild cancer. She refused to consider surgery before seeing me. On her first consultation, I gave her a healthy life-style list of habits, so she can strengthen her immune system to fight that cancer. The list of healthy life style consisted of seven things to do. Let me reiterate.

1. Appropriate amount of exercises.
2. Eat till 80% full and stop, and drink a cup of fluid.
3. Reduce stress with various means. I recommended meditation and music, enough sleep and group support.
4. No sugar or refined foods.
5. Keep same weight.
6. Eat plenty of non-starchy vegetables.
7. Avoid red meat and saturated fats.

That was more than 15 years ago before I knew more to recommend about good foods and bad foods to heal the gut and the immune system. But the above advices were good enough. Six months later in her follow up, she lost three pounds. So she was abiding by all the good life-style habits and lost weight. The CT (computerized tomography) was done before the visit. In the new CT, the golf-ball size carcinoid tumor was gone.

Case #3 is from one of the many books by Dr Andrew Weil, MD (16). It was a case of A.K., a PH.D scientist who worked in a major University. In 1989, A.K. was diagnosed with mixed cellularity non-Hodgkin's Lymphoma. He had been doing a lot of cancer research. He did not believe in modern chemotherapy (he should have, for this disease is curable for most such patients). He chose the "Macrobiotic diet" drawn from Zen Buddhism, "eating brown rice, miso soup, beans, cooked vegetables and sea vegetables. It allowed for no fruits or salads, oils, bread, dietary supplement, meat, milk or milk products, sugar, nor any alcohol". (Very similar to Functional Medicine diets with the exception of good meats and fruits allowed in Functional Medicine diets. The avoidance foods include those avoided in the Paleo Diet).

A.K.'s lymphoma was "controlled" finally. (This may not mean a cure, but maybe even long term control for many years or more. It is possible). Dr Weil recorded another case with ulcerative colitis controlled on similar "macrobiotic diet".

Case #4 is from Dr. Amy Myers, MD's book (18). Case in focus was her father with disabling polymyositis (six similar cases cured in her book plus others). Polymyositis is immune cells attacking one's own muscles all over the body. It is painful and disabling due to extreme weakness and pain. Her dad refused her Functional Medicine treatment of lowering internal inflammation by calming the immune system for five long years with disease getting worse on conventional treatment of steroids and immunosuppressive drugs. These drugs have disabling side-effects when taken more than two weeks or so. Most such patients on conventional treatment are treated year-long, unavoidably, side effects will disable them. Dr Myers' dad had weakened immunity due to the treatment. This weakening was on top of an elderly patients naturally having weakened immunity (unless they exercise and eat the right diet). He had a bout of pneumonia that needed a tube inserted in his chest to drain the inflammatory fluids from the lungs, in the hospital. The whole family gathered there to be ready to bid farewell. Her dad made it out of the hospital that time. Till her father faced a surgery. In this surgery, her dad in his poor health might not make it through surgery. But he got to have this surgery. He backed out of surgery and backed out from conventional therapy and listened to his daughter treating him with very straight Functional Medicine dieting plus very keen and close watch from his doctor. He eventually recovered, free of any conventional drugs for polymyositis. The muscle inflammation was finally gone. The blood test for muscle inflammation that was sky-high, became normal for the first time in five years.

The deterioration on conventional treatment of immunosuppressive drugs is a typical result even for a lot of young and middle age patients. In such cases, I used every other day Prednisone for the patients, not daily. Prednisone is a steroid drug that is immunosuppressive. Every other day Prednisone can avoid almost all deteriorating side effects and yet is equally effective. There are more than ten debilitating side effects for this milder drug. As a medical oncologist, I personally think immunosuppressive drugs, at least the old ones, are worse than chemotherapies.

Case #5 is from Loren Cordain, PhD's book (17). Treating patients with diets is a always cheerful. Here is no exception. The patient was Ms S. She had Crohn's disease. It is similar to irritable bowel syndrome with diarrhea, constipation, abdominal pain and under-nutrition as a result. She lost 45 pounds on Paleo diet, and cured her ulcerative colitis.

The spirit of the Paleo Diet is to eat the foods of the Old Stone Age people. No modern foods like milk, wheat and bread, sugar, salt, processed foods, saturated fats of nowadays (Different than the Paleo period – proteins with less percentage of saturated fats, no toxins, estrogens, growth hormones, antibiotics). Eat plenty of non-starchy vegetables, good proteins, and good fats.

Case #6 described twenty kids with autisms. Got fecal transplants, in effect re-establishing another more normal bacterial combination in the gut, crowded out the old bacterial combination. 83% of the autistic kids were cured. The rest of the 17% improved in symptoms. (This treatment of course has not been proven with big studies).

But now due to the unknown dangers of fecal transplant (one death of more than thousands performed), the FDA only approve fecal transplant for antibiotic related intractable diarrhea, or for research with approval. So fecal transplant is probably out of the question, but it may be possible to change the fecal bacteria combination by eating foods of Paleo/Mediterranean style foods. In other words, avoid bad foods, eat good foods plus minus probiotics of good bacteria. In time, the colon bacteria combination may change. Autism may improve. But please do this under the guidance of a medical or nutritional professional. It would be more effective and safe.

Case #7 was a ten years old kid called Kid P. from Dr Myers book (18). He had rheumatoid arthritis (RA). Conventional medicine made him almost wheelchair- bound for life. He was treated first with conventional medications, he had joint pain and could not walk. One conventional drug after another, only worked for few months before deterioration again. Drugs used included Prednisone, methotrexate (a chemotherapy drug), and then Kineret, a molecular targeted treatment at $1000 per treatment. All failed eventually. Patient was still wheelchair bound.

The father was a business exec and the mother was a physician. They finally had to turn to Functional Medicine. As a result of diet change and good life-style habits pick up. The result was another cheerful case successfully treated by Dr Myers.

At last, the kid was filled with joy that he did not have to take any medications. His parents were apparently happy he could walk again. In his final follow-up visit to Dr Myers, he skipped out of her office, for the last time. I guess his taste-bud cells had renewed themselves in two weeks and he had grown used to the new foods he enjoyed.

Case #8 is almost a psychic mystery story from one of Dr Weil's many books (16). It's a case about Ms K. K. who had aplastic anemia, a very serious disease in which the bone marrow does not put out new blood cells. K. K. had very low platelet because the bone marrow did not put out enough platelets. She could bleed to death during menstruation. So she was treated with hormone ablation to get rid of her menstruation.

Two bone marrow transplants failed to take. She was in isolation room for she had no white blood cells to protect her from any infections. After a very prolonged stay in the hospital and failing treatments, she was sent home to spend the rest of her almost-sure very short life.

She refused to stay home and wait to die. She took up psychic healing. "To do the laying on of hands" and "give blessing". With this power from psychic relaxation, white blood cells came out, and became low normal. Relaxation releasing stress is a very important healthy life-style, as you know. It healed her a little. New studies suggested relaxation can improve the immune cell numbers (white blood cells are part of the immune cells) and cytokines.

She contacted hepatitis B from too many transfusions of blood products. So the psychic devised a special diet for her. " No sugar, no starch of any kind, two eggs and vegetable broths, salads without oil, steamed fish or chicken, one glass of pomegranate or grape juices plus 50% water dilution. (Ah, this psychic had received a message from a higher being in the sky above, and passed it on as the diet –diet similar to Paleo Diet). Hepatitis "got better" and so was the bone marrow which became almost normal.

She was rendered non-fertile with the conventional therapy on purpose. But she wished to have children. So she researched on her own, it seemed, and fasted for one week. In doing this, her gut bacteria might have returned to its primordial combination, because fasting is part of Old Stone Age life. Those good old bugs survived it easily eating whatever available or went into "hibernation", but not the modern bad bugs, I reasoned. The original combination of gut bacteria now can co-ordinate the intricate web of female hormone-interactions, and act on the corresponding organs responsible for hormones in her body. It was really impossible to think medically this could happen. Soon, her menstruation returned.

In the next twenty years, she gave birth to four healthy children.

To sum up -

With these eight cases and thirty-three of my chronic diseases fixed up well just by avoiding bad foods for me, and eat the good foods often, and living the healthy life-styles. Miracles in health care happened. My immune system is strengthened and my chronic diseases went away.

This made me paying more respect to the Father of Medicine, Hippocrates who said more than 2000 years ago, "Food is medicine". It cannot be more realistic that "food is medicine". All the spontaneous diseases, mild ones to fatal cancers, all resolved by switching diets that is mainly vegetable based, with good protein and good fats.

Chapter Forty Two – Chronic inflammation – the real "Silent Killer"

Why is chronic (always there) **inflammation the real silent killer?** – Heart attacks are the most common reason people die of. Next to heart attack are diseases of cancer, chronic lung disease, strokes, Alzheimer's disease, diabetes. All these diseases together with heart attack are responsible for almost all deaths in the world.

Chronic inflammation is the cause for all the above diseases. Chronic inflammation causes and makes the disease worse and worse, till death shall come. This is all done silently but incessantly, by chronic inflammation. Thus the name "silent killer" for chronic inflammation is all but appropriate.

In the past, even though chronic inflammation was there, but no test could detect it, so it was really "silent". It was not possible to detect it, because the inflammation test was done by an insensitive C-reactive protein (CRP). Only in terms of serious whole-body infection like pneumonia, the CRP will go up in the blood test.

So CRP was not sensitive at all. It failed to detect there was a low degree of inflammation that were always there, say, in people with high risk for heart attacks. But now a high sensitivity C-reactive protein (hsCRP) is available. Most people with risks for cardiac events will be shown to have elevated hsCRP. Now silent inflammation can be shown by an elevated hsCRP. It is found in all chronic diseases like diabetes, hypertension, cancer, irritable bowel syndrome. In fact it can be found to be elevated in all of the chronic diseases. And these chronic diseases all can slowly hasten early death before the average life-span of human beings nowadays. These diseases are all due to chronic inflammations which are correctly given the name – the silent killer.

hsCRP is an inflammation marker found elevated in all chronic diseases, the higher the level is, the worse the outcome

hsCRP is elevated in heart diseases, in cancers, in diabetes, in hypertension, in chronic lung disease etc. You name the chronic disease, hsCRP is found elevated. In fact, in patients with heart diseases, the higher the hsCRP is elevated, the higher is the chance of fatal heart attack happening. In breast cancers and lung cancers, the higher the hsCRP, the higher chance death would come. The higher it is in most chronic diseases, it is expected the more violent the course of the disease would be.

Shall we put out this inflammatory fire, say, for the heart?

Yes indeed we should. There came the study called the Canakinumab anti-Inflammatory Thrombosis Outcomes Study, so called CANTOS study. It is a targeted therapy for one inflammatory pathway thought to be particular for heart diseases (there are always multiple pathways doing the same thing), the interleukin-6 (IL-6) pathway. It was measured with the ultra-sensitive inflammatory marker hsCRP blood test. A total of 10,061 people with one heart attack recently were enrolled. The mean LDL was 82 mg/DL, not high. On the average of 3.7 years, results showed hsCRP was lowered on treatment, and cardiovascular events like stroke, heart attack were lowered by 15%. Later, less people were found to be hospitalized for heart failure. But there was statistically significant increase in fatal infections in people given the drug. Nevertheless, this study showed that lowering the inflammatory-fire, would lower cardiac events for sure, though only one pathway was targeted.

But good foods did it better, with studies.

Studies using good foods to stop the inflammatory fire from being set, for the heart

Good foods like MUFA and other good oils (omega-3-like olive oils), olive, green-leaf vegetables in Mediterranean/Plaeo diets were tested against the "low fat" American diet mainly. There are two studies called Lyon Heart Study, and the GISSI Italian study. It was healthy foods (good foods that are anti-inflammatory) against saturated fat fast food American diet with processed, refined carbohydrates (bread, cakes, instant foods that have a lot of HFCS, trans fats, salt and sugar – all inflammatory). The results of comparing good against bad food diets?

1. The Lyon heart study prevented second heart attacks by 70%.
2. The GISSI study lowered deaths from suffering second heart

attacks by 45%.

The above two studies are different than the CANTOS study. The CANTOS study tried to quiet down an inflammatory-fire that was already set, by targeting one inflammatory pathway. These Lyon Heart and the GISSI studies are pro-active, trying to prevent a fire from being set by anti-inflammatory foods that healed a leaky gut, preventing millions of foreign antigens from leaking into the circulation to start whole body internal inflammatory fires. Prevention seems always better than cure.

Prevention of a disease is always cheaper and better than trying to cure

It seems preventing 70% heart attack and 45% death by heart attack by simply eating good foods do a lot of good, was better than by the "targeted therapy" in the CANTOS study of 15% decrease in cardiovascular event. So good eating is so much more effective. Once again it showed that prevention is better than cure. That is, avoid setting the fire is better than trying to put out the fire.

An example of how simple prevention can avoid 150 inflammatory cytokines (cytokines are chemicals of certain function) being made. A piece of thick white bread can activate NFkB, a nuclear factor that once activated, is capable of making 150 inflammatory cytokines, that could take part in a lot of pathways of inflammation. Prevention here is not to eat that piece of thick white bread, and never start the inflammation.

"Food is medicine", the Father of Medicine, Hippocrates, said more than two thousand years ago, it remains true today. A single food contains hundreds of chemicals that could act like medications.

What could be a novo-path for pharmaceutical companies? Give us some prevention drugs please!

Let me be courageous enough to suggest a chance to help control inflammatory diseases, i.e. to help all the people with chronic diseases (billions of people) all over the world. If we can come up with drugs that can quiet down internal inflammation without any side effects, then the population with chronic diseases could use those drugs to achieve super good-health. Internet information exchange is so fast, a lot of common-folks and patients now are aware inflammation is the culprit in heart disease and are really looking forwards to anti-inflammatory drugs that works and without major side effects. Hopefully the new drugs can be broad-spectrum anti-inflammatory against a dozen or so inflammatory pathways, not just one pathway. Biological systems work with multiple pathways all the time, not one pathway only. The block can easily be by-passed by going down another pathway most of the time.

Prevention is better and much cheaper than cure. The cost of healthcare is estimated to match the total US tax revenue by the year 2040, not too many years from now. This won't be like the predictions of "The end of the world is coming in 2040" that would fall flat like a lots of such predictions. The estimation of healthcare cost matching national tax income seems rather real and is not easily solved. But there got to be a start.

In the meanwhile, what can we do?

We know clearly what we should do. It is to avoid bad foods and eat good foods, exercises, get rid of stress, etc. Hopefully too in the long run, some chronic diseases can be wiped out from happening every day. Imagine the money-saving for society, free of the burden of taking care of chronic diseases. It is easier to prevent them than trying to cure some of them just a little. We should know by now, doing this may just help ease the financial burden for our care.

To sum up –

There probably is a good solution for chronic diseases including cancers and heart attacks. It is easier to prevent them with healthy foods and healthy life-styles; as well as help from pharmaceutical companies, to make preventive anti- inflammatory drugs free of side effects. We urgently need that miracle drug.

Chapter Forty Three - Evaluation tools for Herbs

Books, web-sites, organizations to be discussed:
The following are the ones I used as references often. There will be a lot more books listed from the Reference section near the end of the book.

PDR (Physicians' Desk Reference) **for Herbal Medicine** – is published by the same team that published PDR for Medicine reference guides for Physicians. The book based its foundation on the extensive herbal data-base of the PhytoPharm U.W. Institute of Phystopharmaceuticals. It has extensive data on clinical trials of more than 700 botanicals with description of the plant, plant parts used and their chemical constituents and clinical effects. It is followed by clinical trials of different effects and the uses. Then there are the precious sections of precautions and drug interactions and folk uses. It's the first reference I turn to for information. This $400 to $500 book is in almost every public library. Used books can be had for about 30 dollars.

The "Indications and uses" session of each herb mention the approved uses of the herbal drug according to the evidence based research of the German Commission-E, or traditional uses of China, or India etc, and also some unapproved uses commonly deployed. So each "use" was based on research. But as detailed as it practically can be, there is still other uses of the same herbs that is not listed. This indicates the hundreds of chemicals contain in a single herb, serving out many functions that is not possible to be included in a single publication. But it is as detail as the other PDR.

Commision-E – This is a German officially appointed scientific advisory "committee" consisted of twenty four scientific experts who researched or did different studies on herbal medicine in 1978. From 1984 to 1994, the committee published monographs about 380 herbal medications. Since then the monographs have been considered still valid. The PDR for Herbal Medicine used in America and other countries codes the approved uses of Commission-E through the whole book. But updates have been added when necessary.

MSKCC website – This is the Memorial Sloan Kettering Cancer Center website. It has extensive information on herbal medicine, especially when related to cancer management. The information is precise and practical with evidence-based clinical research findings. I was specifically impressed when I look up side effects and adverse case reports of *Echinacea*. The information of *Echinacea* adverse case reports included liver failure and renal failure scared me to the degree I almost dare not even touch the Zinc Lozenges for cold/flu that contains also *Echinacea*. But in a few seconds, I calmed down as I remembered the same scary rare adverse case-reports of any drugs in the medical PDR were just as scary. But I used hundred of those drugs regardless.

Cochrane reviews – It is an organization of a lot of research/academic professionals that produces systemic reviews of primary research in human health care and policies and also independent herbs. It is of very high standard and stringently evidence based. One can look up things in the Cochrane Library on line. (After looking up some herbs with folk remedies that was deemed not enough evidence for this and that. I gave up). They have high standard.

WebMD website – This website offers good practical academic information on a lot of herbal drugs. The descriptions are just detailed enough, objective and practical, and looking up is always rewarding as the site contains a vast amount of information on herbs.

The Herbal Drugstore – By Linda B White, MD and Steven Foster is a gem. It contained information on herbal drugs from the experience of a herbalist (Steven Foster) who has devoted a lifelong career in Herbal Medicine and in herbs. Words are simple and to the point for the real and down-to-earth uses of herbs. Steven Foster spent his whole life in everything with herbs. By the way, he and the legendary American folk song writer are different persons of the same name, but probably of the same statute. I bought one book for $3.5, a used copy from internet. Then I bought another one of the same book from a library sale for $0.25 so I could have one copy of this book for Central Coastal Florida, and one in New York. Its money value is far minimal to the value of the book and other books by Steven Foster and co-authors.

The Supplement Handbook – by Mark Moyad, MD, MPH, is another gem of surprise. It is full of evidence-based information and each agent mentioned stood the practical-use "tested" by Dr Moyad, a urologist well-respected for his herbal and supplements knowledge. The herbs or supplements are classified as "Works" or "worthless", yes, you read it right, "worthless" comment is just that honestly straight. The book is extremely helpful and informative.

But funny enough, *Ginkgo biloba* was classified as worthless for ED, but the herb increased blood flow to the penis, personally I could feel, and as described "effective" in the book "Herbal Bookstore". It actually increased my penile shaft by almost 1.5 mm in diameter when engorged with blood. I brought out this point just to show there is an extreme lack of extensive research on herbal medicine in USA, so there were no validated research reports done on *Ginkgo biloba* on ED, so when practitioners turn to search for this information, one may get none, and that's the end of the information digging.

Generally, most North American herbs have almost never received any meaningful research studies locally compared to say, Europe and its herbs. In fact, *Echinacea*, an original American plant used for hundreds of years by Native American Indians, have most of its researches done in Germany. And in this vast fertile land of USA, there are so many herbs to the envy of herbalists from other countries, few research was done on these herbs in USA.

This is in no way it diminishes the golden value of this precious book that offers so much evidence-based and practical use information on so many supplements and so many diseases.

Part Three

Prevention with New Sciences

Chapter Forty Four - Preventing acute Heart Attacks as much as possible, for real

In new found sciences, what causes heart attack, cholesterol or inflammation?

By now, most people have already known it is not cholesterol that really has caused the heart attack. It is the inflammation. The web carries information fast. Lots of people have been saying the same thing in the internet. It is the inflammation that ended up causing big time heart attacks. What are the studies, and the steps in plaques formation that eventually caused a blocked artery that cut off oxygen to part of the heart muscles leading to heart attack?

Steps of plaque-formation that block heart arteries and cause heart attacks:

White blood cells adhere to the wall of the arteries, because the wall has been changed by the inflammation in the blood. It attracts the white blood cells (that have engulfed oxidized LDL) adhesion as if to mend the wall. The white blood cells start plaque building as part of the repair.

1. The white blood cells secrete chemicals that attract lymphocytes and macrophages to the site. They speed up the plaque building. The plaque incorporates fibrin, platelets, fats and cholesterols. Cholesterols are incorporated whether or not the cholesterol level is high or normal or low.
2. Eventually, the plaque becomes too big. Then the macrophages stop collagen synthesis which was needed for the plaque-building and stabilization. But stopping the supply of more collagens leads to unstable plaques. Under the dynamic force of the currents of the blood flow, the plaque breaks away, exposing the plaque-base. The plaque-base is not normal now, as it has already changed into a very "raw" surface that activates clotting factors and clot formation.
3. The clot eventually blocks off the artery, cutting off blood supply of oxygen and nutrients. The corresponding piece of heart muscles dies. Chest pains occur with the heart attack. In

the absence of inflammation, or if inflammation goes down, any of the above steps will stop. Heart attack may not happen, as the plaque could resolve chemically, like the blood clots that can be dissolved by the fibrinolytic system. But it is clear by this time in the history of heart attack sciences, inflammatory cells are the builders of the plaques and the activators of the clotting system. Therefore anti-inflammation, and not lowering the cholesterol, is the road to lower heart attacks.

What are the studies that lowering internal inflammation can lower the chance of heart attacks?

But the main treatments of heart diseases and heart attacks are, of course, under the care of cardiologists. But in addition, lowering the inflammation will help with conventional treatment to your benefits. Two huge international studies showed lowering inflammation by eating good foods day in and day out for about four years, heart attack rates will go down. These two studies were discussed before in Chapter 42. They are summarized here as follows:
1.   The Lyon heart study prevented second heart attacks by 70%.
2.   The GISSI study lowered deaths from second heart attacks by 45%.

Both studies are comparing Mediterranean/Paleo diets (of good oils like olive, and olive oils, good proteins, and a lot of non-starchy vegetables with lots of fibers) to the American low fat diet. So eating good foods, lowering the inflammation is the way to go to treat heart diseases, along with cardiologists care.

Besides foods, what life-styles help lower inflammation more?

Simply it is the healthy life-styles that help fight heart diseases which are also life-styles that lower inflammations. The life-styles that are encouraged include no smoking, appropriate amount of exercises, a good six to eight hours of sleep, relieving stress, no heavy drinking, but a cup of red wine helps. Besides, the principle of avoiding bad foods like bread, sugar, salt, milk and cheese, saturated fats, trans fats, high fructose corn syrup etc, is of utmost important to lower inflammation. Weight control is also of utmost importance as part of the healthy life-style. Eating to the point of 80% full and then drink some fluid to fill the stomach and stop eating will help control the body weight. When we feel full, we've been over-eating.

The drugs statins can lower cholesterol and reduce heart attacks. But it is not the cholesterol lowering that helped fight heart diseases, it is the anti-inflammatory effect of the statins. Some studies showed the life-styles against heart diseases mentioned above achieve the same benefit as the statins, because good life-styles are very anti-inflammatory too, as strong as the statins and with much less chance for side effects. A lot of people cannot take statins for its side effects, which sometimes can be serious. But nevertheless, it is a good class of drugs in the fight against heart diseases though its effectiveness was due to the anti-inflammatory effects. Cholesterol level has nothing to do with the risk of heart attacks as proven in golden studies.

Exercise as mentioned above, is really the strongest way of lowering internal inflammation as shown in studies. With heart diseases, exercises have to be tailored to the strength of the heart by health professional right at the start. Supervised exercises are part of the cardiac rehabilitation after a heart attack, and American Heart Association recommends regular exercises after a heart attack.

To sum up – **For patients with heart attack before, close follow-up with their cardiologist is the most important. And only then in addition, healthy life-styles and good foods diet are helpful in the total fight against heart diseases.**

Two major international studies have shown Mediterranean/Paleo like diets lowered second heart attacks by 70% and decrease chance of deaths by 45% from second heart attacks, just by lowering internal inflammations. But diet alone is not complete in the fight against heart diseases, healthy life-styles are a necessary part of the fight against heart diseases. Together, they would really prevent a lot of heart attacks and deaths from heart attacks in addition to conventional care.

Chapter Forty Five - Treating and Preventing cancers as much as possible, for real

For cancer patients, can more be done besides conventional treatments?

That was the question I asked of myself all my life. I think finally I figured out what is total treatment for cancer patients. Starting in 1969, I had been caring for cancer patients at first as a radiation therapy technologist, then later as a medical oncologist. I have seen cancer treatments improved a lot, though it has taken some time. At the beginning of my cancer-care career, only 30% of patients were cured. By now, it is only 30% of patients who are not cured. There has been real treatment improvement resulting in a great difference in survival of patients with cancers.

But all along, I know there is more we could do for cancer patients. Like we can ask the patients' body-power for help, yet we haven't. We developed cutting edge targeted therapy aimed at correcting the defect of a single gene. For example for patients with chronic myelocytic leukemia (CML), there was almost no cure before a treatment to correct a single genetic defect was discovered. After the new targeted therapy became available, most patients with CML were cured. But all we were doing was to fight the cancer with drugs. We never tried to help the patients to strengthen their bodies and their immune systems against cancer.

Granted the knowledge and the helping life-style had not been discovered in studies during the dark old days. But it was not the same anymore ten-twenty years before I retired. Lots of hundred-million-dollars population-studies had already proven some life-styles have helped cancer patients survive their cancers a lot better than just getting conventional therapy. So I set out to read more than 500 papers to find what life-styles could help fight cancers. I found quite a few in the late 1990's. I printed those life-styles on a single full 8" by 10" paper and handed it to patients on their first visits. I did not know if those life styles really helps or not in the real world? But in those population studies, about a dozen of the huge studies, all found out the same thing.

For example, exercise can control cancer. It prevented 40% of the cancers. For patients with cancers who do regular exercises, their survival is 50% better, and recurrences (cancer coming back) are prevented by 50%. I said to myself, our state of the art of treating cancer probably will be greatly helped by giving them this single piece of paper, advising those life styles (with tedious explanations in that piece of paper). The list of healthy life-style consisted of seven things to do, in brief again, just as a reminder.

1. Appropriate amount of exercises.
2. Eat till 80% full and stop. (A patient suddenly feasted twice, and each time almost messed up his own aplastic anemia-like disease called myelodysplatic syndrome (MDS). The disease almost got out of control on FEASTING while it had been controlled for 3.5 years without blood transfusions. His case was serious, once out of control, death would come soon. And he learned with me that feasting was dangerous for him.
3. Reduce stress with various means. I recommended meditation, music and group support. (That should include good sleep of 6 to 8 hours a day)
4. No sugar or refined foods.
5. Keep same weight.
6. Eat plenty of non-starchy vegetables.
7. Avoid red meat and saturated fats.

That was more than 20 years ago, I had not yet learned about the new life-styles that help restore the immune system. These "new" life-styles to restore the potent immune system require just one smart move. It is to avoid bad foods and eat good foods to heal the gut and thus the immune system.

First, after I retired and had time to think things through thoroughly, I became convinced that these smart life-styles (listed above) did help. Why not? Those patients with end-stage cancer were supposed to live one year only. But with those life-styles boosting their body-power to control cancer, most of them lived 3 to 5 years. It was no imagination. It was recorded in their medical records. Recently, one of my high-school classmates with lung cancer metastatic to the bones and the liver, and perhaps the brain too on diagnosis, **lived four years by practicing those life styles. Her case-story is in chapter 14.** And for patients with early stage cancers, I hardly remember anybody had their cancers came back. There should be about 20% to 30% cancers coming back. I honestly remembered none. I would be extremely gratified if each new patient on consultation-day, can get one piece of paper like that.

Now with the discovery of chronic inflammation that we can test out by using a new blood test called hsCRP (high sensitivity C-reactive protein), we have proven all the above seven good life-styles are all anti-inflammatory. They all lowered hsCRP. Lowering inflammation is the key to fight chronic diseases, including cancers. For myself, all my 33 chronic diseases are well controlled now just by eating good foods, and more importantly-avoiding bad foods.

Yes, those seven smart life-styles did help save or prolong lives. But really, does avoiding bad foods and eating good foods led to the control of cancers too?

Indeed, the new life-style, plus a few more, does help control cancers. In chapter one, the 3-years old Molly was probably walking on a path to death if we only use conventional therapies. But she healed her guts and her celiac disease, by avoiding gluten. She avoided bread, cookies, cakes and other flour products from wheat. That was it. **Her immune system was restored, and the potency of her immune system at once started killing cancer cells**, and she got turned back to the world of the living. The fatal Kaposi's sarcoma in her right eye disappeared without surgery and or chemotherapy in 2 months.

Are there such cases in cancers that disappeared by themselves? Yes indeed. In one "gold study" of kidney cancers, 5% of the patients with lung metastasis (cancer spread from the kidneys), got the lung cancers disappeared (Most probably by avoiding bad foods, restoring their immune system). But unfortunately most kidney cancers came right back later (Perhaps they were eating the wrong bad foods again and messed up their original potent immune systems again). There are recorded cases of spontaneous resolution of a skin cancers spread all over the body, just to disappear too. These showed when the body-power is tops, cancers can go away. Let's not ignore the body-power anymore. How I wish every cancer patient has the chance to know the above information of avoiding bad foods can probably prevent the beginning of cancers.

My life-long goal might have been realized – to find the cause and do our best to control of cancer

The cause of cancer is due to a deranged immune system that is weakened. Life examples have been provided in this book in different chapters. A weaken immune system allows cancer to grow. So the solution is to restore the potent immune-system for two situations. First situation is for patients with cancers and have been successful treated. It probably is the most important key in the fight against cancer. The restored immune system may stop cancer cells from growing or from starting again. The new immune system probably is strong enough to kill the residual cancer cells left behind microscopically in the body after cancer treatment. The second situation is for people without cancer in the first place. Since the cause of cancer is the weaken immune system. When the immune system is restored by avoiding bad foods and eating good foods, it should be enough to prevent cancer from starting.

And now we know a lot more as how to restore the immune potency of ordinary folks. We may be able to prevent a lot of the cancers in the future when more people have potent immune systems.

Academically, we would not know if all these are true without clinical trials. But fortunately changing diets is up to any individual. If more people can "tune up" their immune systems, get rid of chronic diseases, and subsequently the cancer incidence falls sharply in the coming years, it is as good as clinical trials, isn't it? I honestly believe this will be the case. And I do believe my goal of finding the best ways to control cancer, which I have been seeking for 50 years, has now been accomplished.

I pray to God that messages in this book can reach everybody. Much of my hope could depend on the internet. So please try out the lifestyles and diets. And if this knowledge gained makes a difference to you with your chronic diseases disappearing, I will be grateful if these messages can be spread in the internet. Maybe, and just maybe, I will see a sharp drop of cancer incidence before my time to "float through the tunnel with light at the end of the tunnel", then off the tunnel into the 4th dimension of heaven.

But for now, I am going fishing. My job is done, I believe I have found the best ways to keep the immune system potent.

I never doubt the ways to enhance the immune system I

mentioned in this book. I hope I will live long enough to see if cancer incidence will drop sharply or not. Remember, much depends on you too. I sincerely hope these ways will benefit you.

The complete package of helping to fight cancer

And now with the old smart life-style against cancer that has been proven beneficial in my patients before I retired, now plus the leaning of how to restore one's immune system mainly by "Avoiding bad foods, eating only good foods". Case in focus is myself, I healed my gut, restored my immune system and got rid of the yearly cold. My immune system most probably should be good enough to watch out for cancers that start to appear as "focal foreign objects" and get rid of them in the beginning. I think I have realized my lifelong goal of doing the best to fight cancers, by restoring the potency of the immune system. This is really cancer prevention too.

To sum up – treating or preventing cancers relying on conventional treatments alone is not complete. The patient's body-power from healing their guts, restoring their immune systems (Chapter one), avoiding toxins and plus the seven smart life-styles mentioned in this chapter and this book again and again, should give us a much better fighting chance against cancers. All these good life-styles have good small studies supporting their efficacies, though academically, only large clinical trials will tell if any of these findings mentioned in this book are valid or not.

But the best trials I think are actually for people to do these smart lifestyles, and avoid bad foods, eat good foods in daily lives. And if in a decade of two, the cancer incidences drop sharply, then my goal-of-life of "controlling cancers" would be validated. Even though, personally, I consider my goal has "come true" now.

A more enormous social effect is that these lifestyles and diets can eliminate chronic diseases in the society. And medical expenses will be more affordable. But best of all, everybody will be happier without the same degree of mood swings and depressions.

Chapter Forty Six - Preventing as many chronic
Diseases as possible, for real

New sciences showed most chronic diseases are due to internal inflammation

The internal inflammation is in the blood in our system. It is chronic, meaning it is always there, and not causing any symptoms for us to know. But sensitive blood tests like hsCRP is able to detect the low grade inflammation that is slowly but surely damaging every organs in our body, causing chronic diseases like asthma, seasonal allergy, aging, diabetes, hypertension, heart disease, and even cancer.

The internal inflammation is caused by the chemicals made by immune cells attacking foreign objects circulating in our blood

These chemicals are secreted by our immune cells (white blood cells mainly). They are very potent like hydrogen peroxide, super-oxide etc, designed to kill bacteria dead. But if there are foreign objects all over in our blood. There are so much immune chemicals, our blood would become inflammatory enough to hurt anything coming in contact with it over time. The blood vessels can get hurt, given us cardiovascular diseases like stroke and heart attacks which are chronic diseases. The immune chemicals can attack our joints, we would get arthritis, attack our guts, and we would get diarrheas and so on.

Where do those foreign objects come from?

They came from out gut which is "leaky", so called leaky gut syndrome. In our colon, half the content is dead bacterial parts. In our bowel movement, half the content is dead bacterial parts as analyzed. So we know billions of dead bacterial particles are in our colon. If our colonic surface cells are injured or if the border between neighboring surface cells are open, then it is a "leaky gut". Then millions of bacterial parts can leak into our blood, into our system.

What foods can cause leaky gut?

Leaky gut is not yet an official diagnosis. But this new science will be recognized if most people who avoid the following foods as much as they can and their chronic disease would become better. Then in the future, it will be recognized as a legitimate medical diagnosis. But if avoiding bad foods make us feel good (in about two weeks, it happens), then we do not need it to be a medical diagnosis to do it, because the FDA or Big MED is not going to condemn you from avoiding bad foods and eating good foods.

Gluten is one item firmly established to cause leaky guts in most of us. It would cause leaky gut when the person is sensitive to it. 80% of us are sensitive. Even though only 5% of us would be so sensitive to gluten and develop celiac disease with chronic diarrhea resulting in malnutrition. This is well proven scientifically. Other foods that can cause leaky guts include too much sugar, and night shade vegetables to those who are allergic to them. Night shade vegetables are tomato, potato, eggplants, cayenne peppers. Gluten containing foods include bread, pasta, cereals, wheat flour products, couscous and baked foods. Other possible foods that hurt our gut bacteria are the bad foods like processed meats, cold cuts, deli meats, bacon, hot-dogs. Processed foods usually contain gluten, high fructose corn syrup, trans fats and plenty of salt to make the processed food taste very good. These bad foods can hurt gut bacteria and create leaky guts.

A little bit of the above foods is Ok if you are not sensitive to them (Doctors can test them out). These symptoms are food sensitivities. If the foods make you feel bloated, or feel abdominal pain, causes diarrhea, or constipation. But interesting enough, some good foods can be allergic to some rare people but not most other people. Like sea foods infrequently cause shock and death in some sensitive people, as we rarely can read in newspapers. So make sure you are not allergic to the "good foods" that are new to you before consuming them. Doctors can test that out for you.

Do I believe in avoiding bad food can control chronic disease?

Of course I asked this question as a joke. Thirty-three of my chronic diseases are well controlled just by avoiding bad foods and eating good foods. The one chronic disease that got controlled has been giving me the most pleasure. It is the clear mind I am enjoying and the enlightened mood that it brought. This improved the quality of life so much I simply find it hard to describe. America is a money world. So I won't hesitate to say I feel like a million-dollar man. Or as the value of money goes down with time rather fast, I would say I feel like a billion-dollar man. Hope you feel like one soon.

For USA, then the world (population) to be strong like the "Six-Million Dollar Man", it starts with one – you

Getting rid of the chronic diseases, one feels like "Six Million Dollar Man", a kind of super-human. If each of us gets rid of our chronic diseases, we'll be stronger as a nation, then the world. For this to happen, it greatly depends on spreading the news of these powerful smart lifestyles. Mass communication could get this achieved. But it starts with one, you.

If you try these smart lifestyles, and get healthier, stronger. You naturally will want your loves ones or even other citizens of USA, and the world to enjoy the same benefit, like no mood-swings, no allergies etc. So send it to Facebook, Twitter etc. It will spread to the whole world eventually. It starts with one ---You.

This is a great chance to change the world by the mass communication. Spreading the news can be a good pastime. Yet you will be changing the world.

To sum up – **The best way to control chronic diseases is to use conventional medications like drugs for hypertension, diabetes, or heart disease etc. But much more can be done to control almost all chronic diseases well is simply to avoid bad foods, and eat good foods. I was able to control 33 of my chronic diseases as described in Part One of this book. It has been almost impossible to believe. But it is true as I am living everyday life without the symptoms of my year-round allergy, without pain in my right shoulder, or the wrist. Why? My allergy was cured even without daily Zyrtec, and gone are the symptoms of arthritis, and Carpel Tunnel Syndrome.**

In short, a lot of chronic diseases are curable or controlled well by avoiding bad foods and living smart lifestyles.

If each one of us would spread the smart lifestyles in internet, we may eventually change the world to be healthier and

Part Four

Interesting Matters

Chapter Forty Seven - Should commonly used Medical Herbs be included in Medical Schools' Curriculum and the Paleo/Mediterranean Diet Benefits be taught?

Benefits of Paleo/Mediterranean diets

As I can recall from medical school curriculum in New York, there are hundreds of scientific topics to fit into the short two years of mainly classroom learning, followed by two years of hospital structured leaning (clinical rotations). There is hardly any available time-slot for nutritional learning. But to understand the benefits of Paleo or Mediterranean diets would take not more than an hour of study, because both are very simple to comprehend.

The Paelo diet is mirrored after the foods in the Old Stone Age ancestor's food manual that included wild games they caught (I am glad my restaurant manual is a lot more easy-going). There is a big reason to eat foods like those ancestors did. Theirs and our digestive genes are the same. These genes evolved with mankind for millions of years. The foods that were found at that Paleolithic times (Old Stone Age) about 2 million years ago excluded foods from agriculture and animal husbandry "invented" only 10 thousand years ago. So many of these new agricultural foods probably can present themselves as allergic foods to a lot of people since our genes never saw it before. That included wheat (gluten), milk, and sugar.

So, just avoid milk, wheat flour products and sugar. A lot of serious auto-immune disease will be greatly alleviated or eradicated, as found out by the new breed of Functional Medicine physicians and professionals. Their patients are probably not the typical you or me. They are very sensitive to those foods and breaks out into big time autoimmune diseases like rheumatoid arthritis, polymyositis etc. For the rest of us, however, we can break out into seasonal allergies, arthritis, etc, like the 33 chronic diseases I had. And I need to avoid the new agricultural foods too.

For Mediterranean diet, the main foods are good oils like fatty fish, olive oils, avocado oils, coconut oils, and foods like olives, avocados, and lots of non-starchy vegetables are similar to the Paleo Diet. The cooked vegetables should be more than half a dinner plate (about 40% of the calories) plus good meats and goof fats. Good proteins are like chicken meat, fish meat or sea foods. The Med diet is closer to the Paleo diet

With choices of foods items like that, thousands of Functional Medicine physicians have each healed thousands of people with auto-immune diseases or chronic diseases like allergy or asthma, freeing them from the need of medications and its side-effects. I believe in the power of such practices since I got thirty-three of my chronic diseases cured or well controlled this way.

Chronic diseases care takes a major share of the healthcare dollar, especially if the cost of cancer-care is counted in also. If we don't have to spend that money, we may help lower the cost of health care which is projected to be as big as the US annual taxation income by the year of 2040.

How can we control heart diseases? Just by avoiding bad foods and eating good foods? Yes, Mediterranean diets have been shown in two large international interventional studies of Lyon Heart Study and the GISSI study. Each lowered second heart attacks by 70% and related mortality by 45% respectively.

How can we lower incidence of cancer or prevent cancer in the first place? That needs plenty of studies, not done yet. Maybe we can hold the 3-years old Molly's case up to show as an example of a "pilot study", showing restoring one's immunity was enough to cure a fatal cancer. This point, though needs a lot of study, but by itself, can be taught as an inspiration for future students to develop a career in.

Cardiovascular disease is caused by chronic systemic inflammation with elevated inflammatory markers like high sensitivity C-reactive protein (hsCRP). In the SANTOS Study, a blinded randomized placebo controlled study of more than 10,000 enrollees. It showed lowering hsCRP lowered cardiovascular events. This piece of information is important to emphasize in medical school so the low fat diet can be discarded by medical students.

Cardiovascular diseases are one of the inflammatory diseases with elevated hsCRP test. All other chronic disease, almost all other diseases, elevated hsCRP tests have been shown. Foods have been shown to affect the internal inflammation as discussed adequately in chapter one and most chapters. Isn't this a nice topic to plant the curiosity of future doctors to study and if they find it convincing, to teach future patients and to practice it themselves. We'll at least get some future doctors in constant good moods in their life and ease the hardship that comes with the career in medicine. 4 weeks' trial will probably make them a believer and they will be more enthusiastic to carry out those research works of good foods and bad foods themselves.

Why should avoiding bad foods and chronic diseases be taught in medical school? (For the students own good).

If the spirit of Paleo/Mediterranean diets is taught in medical schools, a new breed of physicians will be well equipped to advise their patients to transform their health, much lowering chronic diseases prevalence in the future, and lowers the cost of healthcare.

Two critical benefits will be apparent at once:

1. Most patients will live a happier life and have a lot less chronic diseases burden on society. The healthcare "dollar" may turn into healthcare "cents". This could lessen the demand of society to "re-organize" Big Med (In reality--Poor Med, thanks to Mr. Flexner).
2. The work-burden will be much lightened on primary care physicians. The heavy burden on primary care physicians at the present time is practically beyond human endurance. Lowering the chronic diseases in patients will lower the future doctors, that is, the medical students, of the future work-load.

   Before I retired, when I realized some hematology or oncology consultation requests were sent to me from the primary care colleagues via the mighty computer network (that cost 6 or 7 billion dollars in the big California health organization I worked in), were initiated at midnight or later. It hurts to know my primary care colleagues were still working in those weir hours.

Herbal Medicines were used since times of the Romans

and the Greeks. How come physicians in the whole world are prescribing them, but not in the US? (We can learn easily)**:**

We can all blame it on the Flexner Report of 1910. Mr Abraham Flexner was a journalist. He was not a scientist, nor was he a medical professional. But he was critical of the medical education in those times for the right reason. I could easily imagine a gun-slinging cowboy of the Wild West era, retired, and could have attended a proprietary medical school and ended up practicing medicine on the street corner in those days, and be our historical colleague? The Flexner Report was written as long as a book, sponsored by the Carnegie Foundation, not a government agency. But it did have a great influence.

Soon following the report, the number of medical schools meeting authoritative requirements set up by AMA to grand MD degrees, eventually the number of medical schools were reduced by more than half in a decade or so. And the quality of medical education had greatly improved in USA. We owed all the excellent quality of care in the US to Mr. Flexner.

But the Flexner Report was nevertheless lacking in the spirit of humanitarianism. I mean herbs takes care of patients as humans, relieving pains, inducing sleeps when needed, and even elevate people from depression. These are humanitarian services the herbs can do. Yet it got excluded because it has no scientific proof of its worth then. Herbal medicine got excluded from medical education because there was no scientific work to back them up. That was, in the year 1910 when Flexner report surfaced. (Women were not allowed to vote then)

But now it has been 110 years later. Herbal medicine has long been scientifically studied for at least half a century

Now there are hundreds of thousands of good studies to back up the herbs. They can be found in say, PDR for Herbal Medicine, on-line and lots of other organizational publications. All constituent chemicals of herbs have been analyzed, their effects studied, and clinically proven. Side effects, drug interactions, and adverse case reports, you name it.

In Europe, nowadays, a medical doctor has to pass the section on Herbal Medicine for the licensing examinations. (Please, not all the herbs! Only the commonly used ones). And in the US take me for example, as result of the American medical education excluding all herbs, at least in 1977 or so, I knew nothing about herbal medicine before retirement. In fact, before retirement, when I was practicing, I got the feeling I should ignore medical herbs because they seemed to me to be useless, just because I was not taught about the herbs. Now I've known about the miracle-like cures I did with the herbs. I looked at my old self with disbelief. How could I have been so ignorant?

Mind you, 40% of the American public is taking herbal drugs. A lot of them are our patients. Could we afford not to learn some common herbal medicine to be truly able to understand why our patients are taking those herbs for? Understanding common herbal drugs is indeed important to a quality good care that we should deliver to patients. This logically should include knowledge in herbal medicine in our future medical education. And there is another reason we should know herbs---the cost consideration (they are cheap), and lowering the healthcare dollars is a must if the students want decent future professional jobs and avoid drastic health-care evolutionary change.

What is it so important about herbal medications?

Nowadays as the money pie for everybody is about the same size like it has always been, but the population has exploded to be much larger. Everybody is getting a smaller share of the money. This limited amount of money would go a longer way if we can lower the cost of medical care. The inexpensive cost of herbal drugs is one of the main ways to lower medical cost. This reason alone would make including herbal drugs a no brainer.

These drugs are at the bottom of the pyramid of cost of medications. For less than a dollar, I had cured my wife's herpes zoster at the rash stage with topical *Tea Tree* oil, avoiding blisters, ruptured wounds, messy scars, and the "hell-fire" like post-herpetic pain. So herbal drugs also can work medical miracles yet are so inexpensive. In this case, *Tea Tree* oil can do what drugs at the top of the medication cost-pyramid cannot do at all, killing the zoster virus at rash stage.

This simply points out herbal drugs have the potential to work miracles, like a few of the drugs at the top of the cost-pyramid. But one drug at the top of the pyramid can buy us hundreds of herbal drugs at the bottom of the cost-pyramid. So if we use herbal medications more, maybe we could do what the Europeans do. Better healthcare statistics than USA, yet at half the healthcare cost. By the way, EU docs are prescribing herbal drugs as well as conventional drugs.

The money spent on a single drug at the top of the cost-pyramid-of-drugs can buy hundreds of drugs at the bottom of the cost-pyramid

Here we are talking about practical things we can use for patients. Targeted drugs with functional monoclonal molecules at the top of the cost-pyramid , save lives and we love to use it. But they required extremely high-tech approach to make and hundreds of millions of worth of clinical trials before approval are hopelessly expensive because the production cost is astronomical. The herbal drugs on the other hand, you can pick up by the trail-side are cheap. Its true value lies in the fact that after thousands of years, they are still around because they have been working. This solid fact is as good as "golden" studies, in all its common sense. Though all popular herbs have their own scientific studies done already by now. Most of the scientific investigations were done outside of USA.

If a few cc of *Tea Tree* oil can cure herpes zoster at the rash stage, it makes sense to use it. To use the *Tea Tree* oil, we have to know a little bit about *Tea Tree*. Is there a problem for future medical students by adding relevant herbal knowledge to learn? No. These are students who are chosen to swallow new information with the greatest ease, no less. But they will be more of super-docs than what they can be. Why not? The knowledge is there, the research is there, listed in PDR for Herbal Medicine, and a lot of other places.

And the great benefit of escaping the "hell-fire" burning pain is there for millions of future patients who will have herpes zoster (shingles). To me, the practice of Medicine with herbs at our disposal is a better and more effective mode of medical practice. Take me for example, I have learned just a bit of herbal medicine, and I have found a couple of medical miracles by herbs in two short years, so I have to say sorry to Mr. Flexner. He should have placed the benefit of the patients in his equation of writing up "the evaluation of medical education" and published his "book" in 1910, not excluding the herbs in USA. He excluded the consideration of the use of herbs in his report, because it was not scientific. Yet now it is very scientific. One just have to read PDR for Herbal medicine, one would agree.

Should "Avoiding bad foods, eating good foods" to restore the immune system be taught in medical schools too? "Yes" is perhaps the appropriate answer.

In Chapter One, we have seen a case of 3-years old Molly cured of a fatal Kaposi's sarcoma by treating celiac disease with avoidance of gluten containing foods. It healed her gut, stop bacterial antigens being absorbed into her systemic circulation, relieving her immune system of millions and millions of immune fights started by the antigens. Her restored immunity regained its true power and got rid of the sarcoma.

The science of avoiding bad foods, healing the guts, restoring the immune system actually consisted of many steps. Each step has been solidly proven scientifically. Take Molly's case as an example. The steps are:

1. Avoid gluten foods. Gluten induces zonulin which opens up intestinal mucosal cells tight junctions. Dead bacterial antigens and other antigens leaked into the circulation by the millions. Starting millions of immune attack all over the body as circulation carries those antigens around, and also locally on the mucosal cells. This vast-scale of immune war generated inflammatory chemicals. (Here, almost all chronic diseases can happen). They are all marked by elevated hsCRP. Those chronic diseases disappeared if the leaky gut is healed. My chronic diseases are cured in a similar way.

    The number of antigens in people with leaky guts far out-numbers the immune cells. The immune system becomes dysfunctional, I think.
2. Healing her intestine which was leaky due to gluten.
3. Her quiet down immune system regained normal function including cancer surveillance and cancer destruction.
4. Attack on the sarcoma began and in two months the cancer was gone.

(As an oncologist, I think this miracle can happen to prevent cancers at the beginning). The above steps have been studied well. For example, gluten inducing leaky gut syndrome has been worked on extensively by clinician/researchers like Dr Alessio Fasano, MD of MGH (Massachusetts General Hospital of Harvard University). The rest of the steps were proven too in hundreds of studies, though mostly in animal studies.

Even if the steps are not proven in humans yet, then these steps still could be considered as hypothesis. Hypothesis can be taught in medical schools too, why not?

The benefit/risk ratio is astronomically askew to the benefit side. If most people practice these good life-style habits and subsequently could eradicate symptoms of chronic diseases as a population. This could lessen the number of chronic-care patients. Healthcare would be a lot easier, and a lot cheaper. This is the most important point in social and preventive medicine as well as in national resources utilization.

There seems to be all things to gain and nothing to lose, by including these topics in the medical school curriculum and perhaps can be included in medical-board examinations too .

In fact, these life-styles are the way of lives in other countries outside USA officially. That is an important reason of why their health statistics are superior to the US and yet only cost 50% as much as in the US. I don't think anyone would consider the US health lifestyle is superior.

To Sum up –

The Flexner report of the year 1910, did improve the quality of American healthcare by raising the standard of American medical education. But the tremendous therapeutic power of herbal medicine, due to its lack of scientific studies in the old days, was excluded in medical school curriculum by the non-medical professional Mr. Flexner. That was 110 years ago. Now there are scientific studies about the herbs. The studies are as detailed as conventional medications. The American patients are at a loss without the herbs. I started learning and using herbs after retirement for several years and found some medical miracles of using herbs (None of the conventional medication can do the same miracles). And yet American physicians are the only ones not using herbs in the world. So now it may be time to consider adding relevant herbal medicine as part of the learning in medical schools. Why is that? Now herbal medicine has been scientifically studied. Most of the studies were done in Europe and outside USA. But they were done, and recorded. Thousands of studies can be found in PDR for Herbal Medicine, or simply, on-line. Herbal mediations are no longer devoid of scientific studies like in the herbal dark

ages of the 1910.

Foods as medicine has cured or controlled thirty-three of my chronic diseases. These tiny bit of knowledge of avoiding bad foods if added to medical school teaching, could lead to physicians giving quick advice that could help cure chronic disease in patients. When the total care for chronic disease is significantly reduced, the cost of care shall be reduced too. And the burden of caring for the elderly would fall about 50% at least (taking care of well patients compared to very sick patients). And follow up appointment for well patients could be once a year instead of several months. This will cut down the patient-load 3 or 4 folds.

Chapter Forty Eight - What would happen to Medicine when Uncle Sam runs out of money?

To be exact, what happens in the year 2040, when the cost of healthcare was predicted to be equal to the total national taxation? –

Well, one choice is Uncle Sam (USA government) can retire or not getting paid, it is definitely not a valid thinking as Uncle Sam is the biggest employee in the world. We know that is not going to happen. Neither would it happen that Dr. Big-Med can just pocket the total national taxation. In reality, Uncle Sam would get the same pay, and print just a limited amount of money more, and pay Big Med (medicine). And Big Med would gradually become Medium Med in the future. Why? Anybody dare do that? In fact Uncle Sam has already been doing that. Medic-Care and Medic-Aid re-imbursements have been so low that it is really not that "believable". Please note, I never said Uncle Sam is mean. But definitely he is a miser. But seriously, there are some ways out, some ways to get medicine out of the hole (that Mr. Flexner dug us into—Science and high tech medicine is astronomically expensive). What change can we make that is good for medicine? There are several possible solutions. Please let me explain.

.It is possible to see even more patients within the same time frame. This is not to turn all physicians into "Six Million Dollar Man" who could accelerate ten or hundred times in his speed of action. It only is possible if most of the patients become very healthy "well-patients" without any chronic diseases. Then in a doctor's visit will be just a few words or reviews for the general health, and a few words of preventive medicine, the doctor-patient visit would be over. It may just take five or six minutes for a proper visit.

.The elderly patients who now have two or more chronic conditions would become more serious as they get older, the visit usually takes at least 15 minutes for a "well-organized" physician, or perhaps would take more than 30 minutes for physicians like me who like to "talk a lot". Now if they have no chronic conditions at all, five minute per visit can be very proper and pleasant.

.How can they be free of chronic conditions, just like magic? Yes, just like magic, I became a healthy old man suddenly free of serious chronic conditions. I adopt the healthy-lifestyles mentioned in this book, and I avoided bad foods, eating healthy good foods as described in Chapter 39. I got rid of 33 chronic diseases like magic. (In reality, have symptoms of chronic diseases well-controlled as to be virtually "free" of the chronic diseases). How do we persuade people to get rid of chronic diseases is important. Patient education is the key. Spread the messages and information in this book is also the key.

.How can Doctor Big-Med become Medium-Med? It is going to be very probable. The Information Technology (IT) jobs are paid as high as physicians now (and work just as hard). And the students capable of doing it will choose IT over medicine just for the time-savings in finishing a professional learning. They would save four years of medical school plus three years for general medical-doc training, and another three years for specialty training (total of ten years). In time, fewer applicants for medical schools are going to happen probably that Doc Big-Med would become Medium-Med in the near future. This brings a big problem to the practice of medicine as physician-shortage has already been a bitter reality even now. So for average patients to be in the well-patient-profiles in the future may help ease the physician shortage.

.Of all memories from life before retirement in my mind, the most bitter memory is always the memory of 5 or more patients waiting to be seen. The thought of too many patients waiting to be seen now even as I am a retired oncologist, the sudden anxiety can fill my mind with fear momentarily. What if I can see 1/3 of the number of patients daily? If that is true, I will gladly come out of retirement anytime. (Yes take me now! I was rated 5-stars). That is not a daydream of a retired man. It can become true. Just look at the numbers. Exercise alone was "proven" in hundred-million-dollars studies like the Nurses Health Study. It has already shown exercises can prevent 40% of the cancers. There, the patient-load would become 60%. In addition, lowering the internal inflammation would bring that down by another 30%, as it is estimated that 30% of the cancers are caused by internal inflammation.

I think the percentage saving should be a lot higher. So finally, if we all advocate healthy life-styles and patients practice it, and lowering inflammation, cancer numbers will, at least theoretically, be cut down by 70% to only 30%.

.How can primary-care doctors be benefited? For patients seen by primary care, when free of chronic diseases, are likely to be seen once a year instead of every three months, since they are healthy enough and do not need so frequent follow-ups. Patients in follow-ups every year instead of every three months making the patient visits drop four-fold. This would ease the physician-shortages now and in the future, forever. So there are all things to gain and nothing to lose to spread the information of smart life-styles.

To sum up – **There is a great chance that future medical practices can be made easier if we advocate to patients the benefits of healthy life-styles and lowering their internal inflammation with new sciences, by giving out hand-out notes for patients' education. If they become free of chronic-diseases then future health professionals would have less health problems to take care per patient. Follow-up once a year would be quite adequate. That cuts down on patient visits three or four folds. It may alleviate the problems of physician-shortages.**

Eliminating chronic diseases diets can also be more thoroughly achieved through public education in colleges, in high schools, or even in grade schools, and most importantly, mass communication through internet. So each of us can help spread the news of how to eliminate chronic diseases and boost the immune system for real. So the new generations growing up would realize that avoiding bad foods will transform one's health. It is easy to prove the habits of avoiding bad foods (for two weeks) will transform health and get rid of chronic diseases. Large scale interventional trials can be done. Since the follow up study is only necessarily to be around four weeks, this type of studies can be very large scale studies and yet is very cheap to conduct, because the time requirement is short. So when will these studies start? This needs governmental interventions and medical world to approve it for their own good.

Once the benefits of avoiding bad foods and eating good foods is proven, meals program in schools can change and the whole generations of young folks will be a lot healthier, and be "good patients" without chronic disease when they grow up and grow old. Their care will be easier and less expensive. Healthcare cost will plummet. All it takes is everybody do their best.

Chapter forty Nine – Paleo/Mediterranean Diets save Lives and the National Budget

Paleo/Mediterranean diets save lives and may save the US national budget too

How can diet save lives? Most of us by now know the answer, The GISSI study showed omega-3 rich diets lowered deaths by second heart attacks by 45%. So diet saving lives is strongly suggested right there. How can it save the US national budget? The answer again is in the diet. You probably remember the Lyon Heart Study that compared the Mediterranean diet against the American low fat diet, the casted away low fat diet in the now infamous food pyramid. (It got two generations of Americans over-weight with chronic diseases numbers increasing at a threatening fast rate). The Med diet prevented 70% of the second heart attacks. This is what would save our bulging healthcare cost. Why? Why not? Let's see what happens here:

1. Yearly non-fatal heart attacks in USA are 1.5 million cases.
2. Each case costs 760,000 dollars. Total cost would then be 11,400,000,000,000 dollars (More than 11 trillion dollars).
3. 70% decrease heart attacks would save 8 trillion dollars a year in the US, provided they all eat healthy foods.
4. Lives saved 1 million 50 thousand, provided everybody knows and all eat healthy foods.

Saving 8 trillion dollars just from one chronic disease, cardiovascular disease. I have "cured" 33 chronic diseases, just imagine the number of dollar saves nationally. It would be hundreds of trillions. No wonder the Europeans are spending half as much as US, and yet have superior health statistics. Their main diet is like Mediterranean diet. This results in less chronic diseases to take care. That is tremendous saving of healthcare dollars. Ok, diets can do it. How about life-styles and herbal drugs, can they save big too?

Healthy-Lifestyles save lives and the national budget too

Take exercises for example of saving lives and money. From

hundreds-million- dollar studies like the Nurses Health Studies (All other such huge studies say the same), exercises prevented 40% of cancers. Just take one cancer as an example for lives-saving and money saving considerations. Colon cancer comes to my mind. It is not even the most common cancer. See what we have here for saving lives and national money:

1. The estimation for new colon cancer per year in US 145,600 cases. Right here decrease of 40% gives us lives saved is around 60 thousand lives free of colon cancer.
2. Treatment for each patient is 70 thousand dollars. Ten billion dollars is the total cost for treatment of all the new colon cancers. Money saved 4077 million dollars.

The lives saved would be more than perhaps 600 thousand. And Money for all cancers prevented would be hundreds of trillions perhaps. Can good life-styles save? So it shows itself capable of saving lives and money right here.

Another example of lifestyle saving money is my knee arthritis cured with the proper exercise, avoiding say, a total knee replacement later in my life. That saved me 49,500 dollars. If everybody like me can get rid of arthritis in their knees with proper exercise early, and in time, then everybody can avoid the total knee replacements. Yearly of 600,000 cases can be avoided. That is 29 billion dollars in savings. Adding the savings all up, we may just be able to cut the cost of healthcare dollars by more than half, better than the Europeans.

Herbal medication saves money too, and can be miraculous

40% of conventional drugs are from herbs. When conventional medication saves lives, there the merit goes to herbs too. No doubt using herbs can save money. If you can pick the herbal plants from the road side, how expensive can it be?

One prime example is the healing of shingles with the anti-herpes herb *Tea Tree* oil. For about fifty cents, I cured my wife's shingles, freeing her from a very likely post-herpetic pain that is described as painful as "Hell-fire". It is extremely painful as reported by my patients. To treat a shingle the conventional way it cost around $100 to $300 just for the anti-viral drugs. You can see the saving here. In this case, it is not the money that counts, it's the efficacy. It is the glorious absence of pain. No conventional drug can totally wipe out the "Hell-fire" pain, the blisters, the ruptured skins holes, the ugly scars. But the Tea Tree oil gets rid of the rash of shingles, and the same day, the disease disappeared (Though the "dead" rash of virus in them persisted for two more days). It is miraculous.

To sum up-

Hundreds of trillions of dollars can be saved with healthy life-styles advocated in this book and using herbs. This might solve the escalating healthcare cost a lot.

Chapter Fifty — Conclusion – A potent Immune System is enough to cure Cancers by Prevention

I still do not believe it is just so simple: The cause and cure of cancers (Provided we know how to keep the immune system potent)

Searching for the cause and cure of cancers has been the goal of my life. It was as if this should be my destiny.

My first job after high school was in radiation therapy (RT) department as a technologist student in Hong Kong. Soon, hundreds of patients with cancers I treated with radiation therapy day in and day out just ended up dying. And hundreds of families lost their loved ones. The images and the faces of the patients and family members haunted me in my mind. These heart-breaking cruelties shaped the destiny for me – to find the cause and cure of cancer. It has been a 53 years pursuit that occupied every second of my mind unconsciously, through years of premedical college courses while working as a RT technologist in NYC, then medical school in NY and beyond.

This obsession never left me all my life as I worked as a medical oncologist/hematologist in New York, then in California. Even after retirement, I ventured into the world of herbal medicine on my own to continue searching. Not finding help there then I turned my attention to health and wellness studies for six more years to search for the answer through dozens of books by learned gurus.

Finally, I saw the light and found out the cause and cure of cancer. It is just hiding under our eyes, and nobody ever saw it. It took me 53 years of search, included ten years of unplanned practical "interventional-trials" with my hundreds of my cancer patients before I retired, The results of the ten years of conventional cancer treatments plus my supplemental advice on lifestyle habits provided miraculous results of survivals. The supplemental advice I gave patients were extracted from the findings of more than 500 scientific and population studies I read on the side. They were proven to fight cancers very well and improved survivals.

These 7 cancer survival tips were the same "immune potency

boosting" tips I have been describing in this book.

What I found is simple. Cancer starts when there is erosion in the immune potency in my patients, either because of lacking healthy lifestyles, or having a poor gut-health that erodes the immune potency. The tips I gave to patients led them to avoid immune erosions that failed them with cancers in the first place. Then the 7 tips restored their immune potency. They ended up achieving survivals that are unbelievable as I will describe below.

What are the results of these practical "interventional trial?" What was the trial?

It never was intended as a trial. It were just healthy lifestyles tips I extracted from hundred-million dollars population studies mainly, like nurses who were treated for cancers but continued their habits of regular exercises, survived 50% better, and prevented the risk of cancer recurrence by 40% etc. All those studies found they can prevent cancers in the first place by 40% too. What were those wonderful results of my "interventional trials"?

The results convinced me restoring the potency of the immune system is enough to prevent cancer recurrences (cancers coming back) which would eventually be fatal

The 7 tips like *regular exercises, keep same weight, avoid sugars, avoid saturated fats, eat plenty of non-starchy vegetables, calorie restrictions, and the release of stress* were all findings from those hundred-million-dollar studies that proved to dwarf cancers. Of the more than 300 patients with breast cancers, for example, the overall recurrence rate is 30% (Early stage with treatment is 5%, without treatment is 9%). So I would expect at least a 100 breast cancer recurrences. But I only remembered 3 patients died of it, and not from recurrences, just from aggressive type of breast cancers that had no good treatments at the time I practiced. Two were young patients with so called Her-2 positive diseases and an elderly patient who was obese with inflammatory breast cancer (which is found usually in younger patients, very aggressive cancer). Otherwise, including the not-so-early-stage breast cancer patients, I remember no recurrence. More than a hundred patients supposed to recur as a historical control, compared to my practical "interventional trial" of no recurrence. This is not "anecdotal case" in any sense.

The success simply means, at the beginning, those hundreds of patients got their breast-cancers and other cancers because they either did not exercise, eating too much sugar, not calorie conscious, or were under lots of stress, etc. Now they realized the page of paper listing those lifestyles and their explanations why it works against cancer was a life-saver for them. They changed their habits. Why not, nobody wants to die. They reversed their erosion of their immune potency, and those remaining cancer cells in them were simply picked up by the now potent immune system for destruction, and there were no recurrences for all early stage breast cancers and other cancers.

When cancers were said to be cured, even for the very early breast cancers, (and other patients with other types of early cancers too), modern tests can detect remaining cancer cells in the blood by a blood test. It is up to the immune system to kill them. What is the basic mechanism of the immune system killing early cancer cells?

Cancer surveillance will kill early cancer for the first time or for cancers remaining after conventional treatments

Now it is well-known and commonly accepted cancer starts after the gene or genes in a normal cell become mutated. As the gene of a cell is mutated, there is some new antigens (structures) appearing on the surface of the cell expressing itself as "Hey, I'm a foreign object". And the immune surveillance cells will label it for destruction by the immune system. So if the immune system is normal, it will be potent enough to destroy the new cancer cells. Cancer will only grow if the immune system potency is eroded.

While immune potency is restored by avoiding immune erosion habits, it can kill cancers.

A restored potent immune system will kill cancers

Remember the cases mentioned in chapter one? Molly the 3-years old girl had a fatal Kaposi's sarcoma in her right eye, because of immune erosion by her celiac disease causing the leaky-gut-syndrome, eroding her immune potency. But avoiding foods containing gluten, she healed her leaky-gut and the Kaposi' sarcoma disappeared from her right eye. My patient with carcinoid cancer had it eliminated from her left lung. And others patients with cancers spontaneous disappeared were all probably related to restoring the immune potency. There is more proof in the general population that a normal and potent immune system is all it takes to prevent cancers.

80% of the population has no cancers life-time

They are lucky, we used to say. But now, it can be explained in what is the truth, I think. They simply have normal immune-systems that are capable of cancer immune-surveillance. There are 5000 mutations per person per day on the average, some of which can lead to early cancer growth, were all picked up by the immune system and killed in those 80% of the population that never have cancers.

That has nothing to do with luck. That shows all the glory of the potent immune systems.

Concluding remarks

I dare not believe it is just so easy to cure cancers by preventing cancers in the first place or preventing cancers from coming back. But evidence from findings of those population studies and my own God-given practical "interventional study" and its good results have convinced me the cure of cancer is just possible by prevention with lifestyle changes. These changes we all can make.

With these said, my tons of mental burden to find the cause and cure of cancer, should be lifted from my shoulder. I have been feeling like a free man for the first time in my adult life for almost a month by now. I never fell free till what I have to do is done. Now it's done.

But lots of swimming, sailing, and fishing have to wait. USA is still in the lock-down mode for the Coronavirus pandemic of 2019-2020.

List of reference books and websites
Websites:
1. WebMD
2. Memorial Sloan-Kettering Cancer Center MSKCC
3. Cochrane Reviews
4. Wikipedia
5. Google Scholar
6. NIH articles when needed
7. Google Search

Reference books (Listed at random)
1. PDR for Herbal Medicine.
2. LifeExtension – Disease Prevention and Treatment, 5th Ed
3. The Herbal Drug Store – Linda B. White, MD, Steven Foster
4. The Supplement Handbook – Mark Moyad, MD, MPH, With Janet Lee
5. Microbiome Solution – Robyme Chutkan, MD
6. Autoimmune Fix – Tom Obryan, DCCCN,DAC, BN
7. Herbal Antivirals – Stephen Harrod Buhner
8. The Clever Gut Diet – Michael Mosley, MD
9. The FastDiet – Michael Mosley and Mimi Spencer
10. Ultra Metabolism – Mark Hyman, MD
11. Gut Makeover – Jeannette Hyde
12. Food Can Fix It – Mehmet Oz, MD
13. Nature's Medicine – Steven Foster and Rebecca L. Johnson (NGeo)
14. Natural Health, Natural Medicine – Andrew Weil, MD
15. Healthy Aging – Andrew Weil, MD
16. Spontaneous healing – Andrew Weil, MD
17. The Paleo Diet – Loren Cordain, PhD
18. The Autoimmune Solution – Amy Myers, MD
19. The AntiOxidant Miracle – Lester Packer, PhD, Carol Coleman
20. The Inflammation Syndrome – Jack Challem
21. Cavewomen don't get Fat – Esther Blum, MS, RD, CDN, CNS
22. The Probiotics Revoultion – Gary B Huffnagle, PhD with Sarah Wernick
23. Hormone Reset Diet – Sarah Gottfried, MD
24. Master Your Metabolism – Julian Michaels
25. The Human Microbiome – Rebecca E. Hirsch
26. Natural Antibiotics and Antivirals – Christopher Vasey, ND
27 Make Peace with Fat – Mihaela A Telecan, DVM, RD
28. The Micronutrient Miracle – Jason Calton, PhD, Mira Calton CN

29. Mental Health Naturally – Kathti Kemper, MD
30. Eat Fat, Get Thin – Mark Hyman, MD
31. Atkins for Life – Robert C. Atkins, MD

32. The South Beach Diet – Arthur Agaston, MD
33. "Peterson Field Guides – (Eastern Central) Medicinal Plants – Steven
Foster/James A. Duke
34. Mayo Clinic Book of Alternative medicine
35. American Cancer Society – Complete Guide to: Complementary & Alternative
Cancer Therapies
36. Who is not afraid of Cancer – James C. Shum, MD
37. Run, Run, Run, run away from Cancer - James C. Shum, MD
38. Preventing Cancer Recurrence – James C. Shum, MD

Index

A

O

Oregano essential oil 73, 147, 150, 151, **154,** 155, 156
Oropouche Fever 155
Osteoarthritis 53, 65-71
- And stem cells **67**

P

Paleo diet 27, 85, 128-129, 159, **243,** 244, 245
Peppermint essential oil 139
Probiotics 48, 110, 218, **231**
- And bladder cancer
- **As chemical factories for us** 236-238
Prostate specific antigen (PSA) 50, 58, 59, 131, **158-160**
- Lowered by diet 159
- Lowered by lifestyle 159
Psoriasis 58, 148, **150**
- And *Aloe vera* 151
- And *Oregano* essential oil 150

Q

Quercetin 78, 217

R

Respiratory virus pandemic (of 2019-20200), 14-17, 24, 79, 99
- Respiratory virus pandemic and dangers of immune-
  compromisation 36-38
Retinal bleeding 123-126, 180
- And other herbs 124
Retinal bleeding continues
- And supplements

S

Sambucol 17, **18**

T

V

Z

www.ingramcontent.com/pod-product-compliance
Lightning Source LLC
Chambersburg PA
CBHW031052250726
48655CB00004B/1400